Training Trances

Multi-Level Communication In Therapy And Training

John Overdurf & Julie Silverthorn

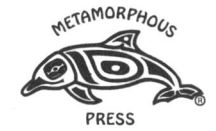

Metamorphous Press
Portland, OR

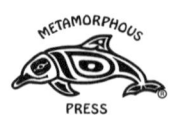

Published by
Metamorphous Press
P.O. Box 10616
Portland, OR 97210-0616

All rights reserved. No part of this book may be utilized in any form or by any means, electronic or mechanical, including photocopying, recording, or by any information storage and retrieval system, without permission in writing from the authors.

Copyright © 1994 by John Overdurf, C.A.C. and Julie Silverthorn, M.S.
Copyright © 1995, Third Edition, by John Overdurf, C.A.C. and Julie Silverthorn, M.S.
Editorial and Art Direction by Lori Stephens
Printed in the United States of America

Overdurf, John, 1957-
   Training trances : multi-level communication in therapy and training / John Overdurf & Julie Silverthorn.
     p. cm.
   Includes bibliographical references and index.
   ISBN 1-55552-069-3
   1. Hypnotism—Study and teaching. 2. Neurolinguistic programming—Study and teaching. I. Silverthorn, Julie, 1958-. II. Title.
   RC497.094   1996
   616.89'162—dc20   95-43393

ii

Table of Contents

Foreword by Tad James   *vii*
Introduction   *xi*

Chapter 1
Two Minds Defining Trances   **1**

Chapter 2
What Do Driving And Garages Have To Do
With Intention And Trance?   **15**

Chapter 3
Structuring Trance Inductions, Naturally   **41**

Chapter 4
Dissociating Functions—Communicating Possibilities   **61**

Chapter 5
Catalepsy: Giving Your Trancework A Healing Lift   **81**

Chapter 6
Hypnotically Skillfull   **103**

Chapter 7
The Hypnotic Interview:
The Inner View of Trans-Formation   **127**

Chapter 8
Posthypnotic Suggestion: How To Trans-fer The Learnings   **149**

Chapter 9
Constructing Stories: What Is A Metaphor, Anyway?   **165**

Chapter 10
Metaphorical Intervention: Is It Real Or Just A . . . ?   **183**

End Notes   205
Appendix   218
Bibliography   228
Index   232

Dedication

to the spirit of Milton Erickson

to the spirit that lives as his work

to the spirit that changes us

to the spirit of all that is

to the Spirit

Acknowledgments

We would like to thank the following people who participated in our Hypnosis II seminar held in September, 1993 upon which this book is based (in alphabetical order):

Brantley Alexander	Jacqueline Paltis
Lee Bowers	Dot Parker
Don Hinkley	Patrice Perillo
Spike Humer	Char Saji
Robert Leichtman	Paul Talley
Dottie Lownes	Tempa Wadsworth
Christopher Minch	Sam Weider
Meredith Mueller	Dave Wolf
Coleta Nova	Cindy Zollman
Dan Outcomer	

We would also like to thank everyone who participated in the following trainings for their support and patience as we were working on this project:

1994 Practitioners of NLP—New Zealand
1994 Accelerated Practitioners—Lancaster, PA
1994 Hypnosis II—Lancaster, PA
1994 Practitioners of NLP—Lancaster, PA
1994 Master Practitioners of NLP—Lancaster, PA

Special thanks go to Bob Braem and Cindy Zollman for asking, "If you are doing Hypnosis I, when are you doing Hypnosis II?" Without that question, this book may not have been a reality.

Special thanks to Julie and Nick Jarman for all their assistance and friendship. They made sure we had all the necessary provisions to keep working on this while overseas for a month.

Special thanks to Harold and Violet James for their interest and enthusiasm in working on this project. Their editorial assistance was priceless. We are very grateful for all their contributions seen and unseen.

Special thanks to Brantley Alexander for his desire to be part of this creative process. His expertise in editing was invaluable. We truly appreciate everything he has shared with us over the years.

Special thanks goes to Dave Soehren for his genius and creativity in designing the manuscript cover. We were honored to have his work as the visual metaphor for the early editions of *Training Trances*. Thanks also to Ed Sisler for his enthusiasm and dedication to the project.

Special thanks to Tempa Wadsworth for being who you are—with all your enthusiasm and excellence. Thanks for assisting us in getting our message out.

Special thanks to Donna and Ralph Upson, the "real" Neuro-Energetics "trans"-scribers, for all they've done for us during our years of working together.

Special thanks to the fine folks at Metamorphous Press, especially Lori Stephens, Senior Editor, for the elegance, clarity and creativity she contributed to this work. We truly appreciate her valuable time and suggestions.

Special thanks to Ron Klein for being one of our mentors on this path. Your guidance and support was more valuable than you could know.

Special thanks to Ardie and Tad James for their friendship and most of all their unconditional support. Also thanks to all our very good friends at Advanced Neuro Dynamics for being some of the most "decent" folks we've ever had the pleasure of working with. Thanks to Donna Morabito for asking about this project and encouraging us past the wall.

Special thanks to Agnes and Ivan Silverthorn and Jeanne and the late Anthony Overdurf for making it possible for us to be living this lifetime.

Finally, a very special thanks to Milton Erickson for being who he was and so much more.

Thank you all for sharing your magnificence and most of all for believing in us.

Foreword

by Tad James

When I first saw Hypnosis demonstrated in a training environment, I was amazed at how deeply people went into trance with only the assistance of a trainer "just talking" to them! When I looked further, I noticed that the "training trance" was as deep as any therapeutic trance I had ever seen. As I began to develop my own training and teaching style, I realized that the use of trance in training was an essential part of learning. I also recognized that trance was a normal reaction in the training environment and that untrained trainers were also eliciting trance from their students and not recognizing it. I decided that I wanted to use trance purposefully in my trainings, not randomly as others had, so I asked myself, "Who would be the best model for this?"

Erickson's approach

Milton Erickson's[i] hypnotic approaches are extremely useful in the training context because they do not rely on formal trance inductions. Erickson was very conversational and natural in his approach to Hypnosis. It was his view that trance was about *learning* to go into a trance, but what if *all* learning was about trance?

Learning and recall are to a great extent the result of unconscious processes, especially when storing and retrieving information. Therefore, learning is facilitated and enhanced by communication with the Unconscious Mind. For years, studies have indicated that hypermnesia, which is increased memory and recall, is possible in trance. Trance, used in a training context, will therefore facilitate learning and recalling information.

Trance is also very useful in the therapeutic context because it depotentiates the conscious mind. Erickson typically framed clients' problems as a function of their conscious processes and the resources as a function of the unconscious processes. He believed trance was the optimum state for getting in touch with the internal processes which would provide the solution for the clients' problems.

Facilitating unconscious communication

Why is the facilitation of unconscious communication important in both training and therapy? As information is learned, it goes through our conscious

vii

filters and once learned, it is stored at the unconscious level. For example, think of all the phone numbers you know. Think of your home phone number. Can you say it to yourself? Good. Now, where was your home phone number before you said it to yourself? It was stored at the unconscious level! Obviously, if it was stored at the conscious level, you would have to consciously remember it all the time so you wouldn't forget it.

Fortunately, our Unconscious Mind stores what we have learned and facilitates the recall of that learning. Since that is the case, the processes of learning and recall are greatly facilitated by direct communication with the deeper levels of the mind, with the Unconscious Mind. In this way, learning and recall become more profound.

So how does the trainer and therapist strategically utilize unconscious processes to benefit students and clients? *Training Trances* answers this question by providing an excellent summary of effective techniques and procedures for facilitating learning and unconscious communication in both training and therapeutic environments. It is an important addition to the current literature in the field of Hypnosis and it is the first book, to my knowledge, which discusses trance from a Trainer's point of view. Also, it is written as an example of hypnotic literature and can be read on multiple levels: from the trainer's, therapist's, or client's point of view. Along with this process information, this book provides unique and expanded insights into Erickson's work, which are invaluable to the practicing hypnotherapist.

Julie and John developed this information from their considerable experience in Hypnosis and training. I met them at one of our earlier Trainer's Trainings and recognized the level of personal commitment they had to working with the Unconscious Mind. They rapidly integrated this commitment into their own individual training styles and joined me on the teaching staff of our Annual NLP (Neuro-Linguistic Programming) Trainer's Training, where the use of trance is a central theme. Today, they are two of the absolutely best trainers in the field of NLP and Hypnosis.

Where to from here? The future of Hypnosis and trance

As we look back on the 1990s from the perspective of several decades in the future, we will look back on this era as the time when science verified the mind-body connection. Previously, science could say that "Hypnosis is just in your mind." Quantum biologist Deepak Chopra[ii] and many other researchers are now certain that neuro-transmitters, which were previously thought to be only in the brain, actually have contact with every cell in the body. With the capacity of neuro-science to measure the presence of neuro-transmitters, we now know that mind has the ability to contact and, therefore, to affect every cell of the human body. The effect of mind in the body is obvious to many researchers and clinicians today. What is not so immediately obvious is that Hypnosis, and other processes that contact and work with the Unconscious Mind, have the greatest chance of making a difference at the physical level.

Historical uses

As early as 1860, Pierre Janet and Alfred Binet[iii] demonstrated that dramatic alterations in physiological functioning could be produced using hypnotic and other similar techniques. Researchers in the late 1800s were creating diseases and other physiological symptomology and then taking them away using Hypnosis. With Freud's rejection of the science, Hypnosis fell into disuse among the psychological and medical communities. For almost a hundred years, many people in psychology and medicine looked upon Hypnosis with disdain. Today, that unfortunate oversight is being corrected as practitioners and researchers alike begin to look again at the incredible potential that Hypnosis has for learning new ways of being mentally and physically healthy. In this context, Hypnosis may be the most valuable subject you can learn.

Learning and recall

Imagine being able to learn, remember, and recall anything that you want! Being able to heal unwanted mental symptomology.
Being able to heal unwanted physical symptomology. Being able to change any physical condition that you have. All these are facilitated by Hypnosis and by communication with the Unconscious Mind.

Hypnosis revival

As we look forward to the next millennium, I believe the revival of interest in Hypnosis and unconscious processes will move the science of the Mind to new understandings and to new discoveries about the full extent of mind-body communication. I see an exciting time ahead, because the limits of what the human being is able to do both mentally and physically are being explored and expanded.

Personally, I have been interested in exploring those limits for a long time. Over the past several years, much of our exploration has taken place as we developed and refined our Time Line Therapy® Trainings. This will continue, as will the exploration done in conjunction with the Doctoral program in Clinical Hypnotherapy at the American Institute of Hypnotherapy. It is time to expand the mental and physical limits of human capability through trance and communication with the unconscious mind. *Training Trances* is an excellent example of what is possible when communication with the Unconscious Mind *goes deeply* . . .

> Tad James, M.S., Ph.D.
> Certified NLP Master Trainer
> Developer Time Line Therapy®
> President, American Institute of Hypnotherapy
> President, Advanced Neuro Dynamics

---

i   Milton Erickson, M.D. was, until his death in 1980, one of the world's foremost hypnotherapists. He was probably responsible for most of the indirect permissive hypnotic techniques used today. Any book by Erickson and Rossi, or Erickson and Zeig, is a good place to start your investigation.
ii Deepak Chopra, *Quantum Healing*, Bantam Books, 1989.
iii Peter Brown, M.D., *The Hypnotic Brain*, Yale University Press, 1991.

Introduction

What is the purpose of *Training Trances*?

If you're reading this book, it probably means that you have been studying Hypnosis in some form and you want to learn more. This book represents an aspect of our current understanding in a very small area of Dr. Milton Erickson's work. Unfortunately, we never met Dr. Erickson in person; therefore this represents our interpretation of his techniques from his published writings, videos, and audios. Only he (or probably, more specifically, his unconscious mind) would know how closely we truly are to understanding what he intended.

We can say that the spirit of his work has touched us deeply and has been a constant inspiration to us in our work and our lives. It's this spirit that led us to the many discoveries and insights which resulted in this book. One of the most profound realizations which we had throughout our years of training and research in this area called Ericksonian Hypnotherapy is that Erickson never did "Ericksonian Hypnotherapy." He did whatever he believed was necessary at the time for his clients to change. His pragmatism enabled him to work equally effectively with a broad spectrum of clients—from psychotics to psychiatrists. He left behind a legacy of indirect approaches which broke new ground in hypnotherapy. However, despite his reputation for being indirect, he could also be very direct and traditional in his hypnotic approach. A few years ago, one of our colleagues casually mentioned that in all of his travels he had found very few people who were trained in Ericksonian (indirect) techniques **and** who were comfortable producing the classical hypnotic phenomena. We considered the merit of his comments and, as a result of subsequent discussions, developed this training. Our primary objective in both the training and the book is to blend Ericksonian and traditional models in a manner not previously documented.

How did *Training Trances* develop?

We developed this book from transcripts of a four-day workshop conducted in September 1993. The participants had a previous understanding of rapport and hypnotic language patterns, along with a working knowledge of NLP and Hypnosis. We are presupposing that the reader also has a similar knowledge base. Additionally, all of the participants had previously attended at least one seminar with us, so rapport and trancework could deepen very quickly.

As you might expect in a small, intimate training, the most significant communication was, at times, nonverbal. There were times when we may have said little or nothing, and yet everyone understood what we were communicating. Some of the most powerful communication which occurred between the participants and trainers could have been in the form of a look, a raise of the eyebrow, a change in voice tone, a smile, a nod, or some other kind of gesture. Our challenge in writing this book was to preserve the "training atmosphere"; so we edited the audio transcripts, minimally in some places and considerably in others, to convey the same or similar message to you, the reader.

The text of the book makes few references to the fact that it is a book. Rather than say, "In the next chapter," we may instead say, "In the next section," or "Later on we'll be discussing . . . ." Also, questions from the participants are included in the transcript when they provide an opportunity to demonstrate skills being taught or when the questions address important areas for expanded commentary. The references and the inclusion of the questions are intended to convey the spirit of the training and to make the book a "Training Trance."

The design of the book closely parallels the design we chose for the training itself. The training design incorporated hypnosis extensively in direct and, more often, in indirect ways, in the presentation of content, demonstrations, group inductions, and exercises. During the workshop, participants were continually going in and out of various levels of trance. Often in a training context, one of the most opportune and subtle uses of positive, indirect suggestion can occur during the presentation of the factual, more "left-brained" content. During these times, the audience is consciously absorbed, paying attention to the content, thus making it easier for us to provide suggestions which communicate directly with their unconscious minds. Over the course of a training there is a multitude of opportunities to make suggestions about how much learning or transformation is occurring. As you read this book, you may notice these types of suggestions. (If you don't, that's okay. It just means these suggestions were included in your unconscious learning!)

During the "live" training, a significant amount of learning occurred during the exercises. The participants usually did the exercises in dyads or triads, giving each the opportunity to experience being the client, the hypnotherapist, and perhaps the observer. The exercises from the training are included in this book to provide the context for how trance is taught. These protocols are also useful for the reader who may choose to practice these skills. Additionally, the sequencing of the exercises in the book is the same as in the workshop. Earlier exercises are purposely sequenced to build skills and install formats which are used later in the training; the later exercises focus on problem-solving and therapeutic interventions.

How is this book written?

This book has been written, loosely speaking, holographically. This means that, in most cases, any section you read will be representative of the whole. Each section of the training contains within it the basic presuppositions of the entire book. On a second level, <u>how</u> we teach each section will be representative of <u>what</u> we are teaching in the training. On a third level, <u>how we have written</u> each section is representative of <u>how we are teaching</u>, which is representative of <u>what we are teaching</u>. The book is an example of multi-level communication conveyed through the single medium of the written word.

One of the challenges of writing a book about Hypnosis, which occurs within the training context, is the choice of language types or styles. When using hypnotic language there are numerous occasions when we may purposely violate grammatical rules to create certain effects which produce trance. Generally speaking, these violations are made with the intention of producing ambiguity. For example, you may notice our tendency to use the second person extensively and often generically. We might say something like, "When <u>you</u> talk to your client, you want to hold the internal representation, '<u>You're</u> a great hypnotic subject.'" We do this to create a linguistic context within which we can provide direct suggestions (i.e. "You're a great hypnotic subject") to the audience in the seminar or even, dare we say, to you the reader! Other similar examples include incomplete sentences and sentences which do not logically follow; these can be readily observed in a number of the inductions. Let us assure <u>you</u> that we are aware of the language we use, and more than that, our use of it is purposeful. Whenever possible, we have modified the text to be grammatically correct, particularly when what we say is not intended to be hypnotic language.

We utilize a number of conventions in this book to make it easy to read and to identify easily the different levels of communication. So that the reader may develop a familiarity with these different levels of communication, we are using specific type styles. For the sake of simplicity and consistency, we have made four variations in the type style: plain text, **bold**, *italics,* and ***bold italics***.

1. Plain text—primary content of the training or text; or for lengthy trance inductions which are clearly labelled.

2. *Italics—interspersed suggestions with voice analogs.*

3. **Bold face—headings and/or special hypnotic emphasis.**

4. ***Bold face italics—special hypnotic emphasis within a trance induction.***

Secondly, along with the traditional headings at the beginning of the sections, we also use graphics to identify easily and unconsciously what you are about to read:

Editor's Notes Demonstration

Induction Exercise Procedure

You may notice as you read some of the early chapters that we describe important nonverbal behaviors which accompany the dialogue. (These will be found in parentheses.) As you read succeeding chapters, we gradually phase these out. Our expectation is that you will start to fill in your own ideas and hypotheses about the accompanying nonverbal behavior, as you learn and understand the models presented.

You may notice that this book includes footnotes. We have elected not to use the standard APA (American Psychological Association) format for footnoting, as we believe it breaks up the flow of the "training." Instead we use standard footnotes with content notes. The latter are valuable in cases where there is pertinent "left-brain" information or explanations which supplement the training. There is plenty of information in the content notes for trivia fans and they (yes, the content notes and probably the trivia fans, too!) may be found in the back of the book.

Each chapter begins with the "Editor's Notes." In these notes we delineate the purpose of the chapter, highlight certain points, make clarifications, and/or ask questions to frame the chapter for easier reading. These notes vary in length depending upon the amount of framing necessary for the reader to experience unconscious familiarity with the subject matter. In the chapters where direct framing occurs, the notes will be minimal. If you are an experienced trainer or practitioner of hypnotherapy, you may want to consciously skip over the Editor's Notes.

We use a standard training design throughout much of the book. The text of each chapter will usually begin with some preliminary information about what will be taught, and "why" it is important to learn that material. Answering the question "why" creates intention and motivation to learn in the audience. Also in this phase of the presentation we may use stories, analogies, and other conventions to format or prepare the unconscious mind for the information which will follow, so it is more easily organized, assimilated, and integrated. Here's an example of what we mean by formatting: Let's say we have a large area that we want to use as a parking lot. We want to optimize our resources. We want to make it easy to park the largest number of cars possible while maintaining some order. To accomplish this, we draw lines for the park-

xiv

ing spaces and put up signs for different sections, so the drivers know where to go in the parking lot, so they aren't wandering around creating traffic jams. Formatting ahead of time makes it easy to know how to drive through the parking lot, where to park, and where to go when we're ready to use the car again.

In each section, we frequently do a covert demonstration of the skill for the audience and one which is slightly less obvious for the reader. The purpose of a covert demonstration is to create a sense of familiarity with the information presented later. After the covert demonstration, we do an overt demonstration of the skill being taught, an exercise to integrate the skill, and a discussion at its conclusion to handle questions and assist in transferring the skills to future contexts.

What is included in *Training Trances*?

In Chapter One, "Two Minds Defining Trances," we begin with a discussion of the underlying concepts about the nature of the conscious and the unconscious minds and trance. We highlight Dr. Erickson's most famous notions and corroborate them with more recent research. These recent sources are worth exploring, particularly if you are going to practice or teach hypnotherapy. In this chapter, we set the major frames for the entire book.

What do driving and garages have to do with intention and trance? You probably never wondered about this before, but if you are wondering now, you'll want to read Chapter Two. In this chapter, we start with a *brief* explanation of direct and indirect suggestion. We confine our discussion to when and how both are useful. There's also a double induction to set up the training along with a discussion of Erickson's utilization principle, which is one of the hallmarks of his work.

Chapter Three, "Structuring Trance Inductions, Naturally" and Chapter Four, "Dissociating Function—Communicating Possibilities" cover basic approaches to trance inductions. Understanding these will provide a framework for understanding any traditional or scripted induction. By the way, if you really want to learn how to do these, make sure you do the exercises. Practicing them will insure a direct experience of the suggestions and will install the abilities necessary for the formats presented in subsequent chapters. They're also lots of fun!

Chapter Five, "Catalepsy: Giving Your Trance a Healing Lift," covers the elicitation and utilization of catalepsy. It includes three more inductions utilizing catalepsy and our ideas on how catalepsy can be used in changework and physical healing.

Chapter Six, "Hypnotically Skillfull," surveys all of the other classic hypnotic phenomena. We focus on and expand upon dissociation, analgesia/anesthesia, amnesia, and deep trance identification. You will learn the "how to's" as well as where and when to use them.

Chapter Seven, "The Hypnotic Interview: The Inner View of Trans-formation" integrates the first six chapters into an interview format. The interview steps include: gathering the initial information, utilization, trance inductions, elicitation of hypnotic phenomena, changework, and posthypnotic suggestion. This hypnotic interview is based upon our modeling of a number of published therapy interviews conducted by Erickson. This is an extremely versatile and flexible interview.

Chapter Eight, "Posthypnotic Suggestion: How to Trans-fer the Learnings," deals exclusively with . . . , . . that's right . . . . . . posthypnotic suggestion. In this chapter, we outline a basic protocol which we noticed Erickson weaving through a number of his interviews. This outline also corresponds with the experimental research he conducted in the area of posthypnotic behavior.

The final two chapters, "Constructing Stories: What is a Metaphor, Anyway?" and "Metaphorical Intervention: Is It Real Or Just A . . . ?" are our interpretation of how Erickson seemed to use therapeutic metaphor. This structure ties together all of the components discussed in the previous chapters and is a delightful way to work. Chapter Ten includes our version of the Hypnotic Dream Induction, which is a sleeper and that's fine with us. We hope you enjoy it.

What is the best way to read *Training Trances*?

Training Trances is written as an example of hypnotic literature. Since it's a book about hypnosis, we decided to incorporate hypnosis into our writing style. Readers who have a hypnosis background may notice that some of our references are more obvious and explicit than others. The text styles and icons indicate the most obvious segments. Just for the reader's enjoyment, we have included hypnotic language patterns which we did not label. You may find it an enjoyable experience when you discover them.

As you're reading this book, you may notice from time to time that your mind may wander. You might initially think that you're not staying focused or not absorbing the information. While it is important to us that you increase your conscious understanding of hypnotic techniques, it is equally—if not more—important that your unconscious mind experience the patterns used. One of the primary purposes of indirect hypnotic language is to stimulate associations. Therefore, unlike other technical books which you may have read, it is perfectly acceptable and even encouraged to let your mind wander while you read this book. Making meaningful associations will make reading this book a valuable experience for you.

It has been our experience that when reading any good book, we make new connections and develop creative ideas from the stimulation provided by the particular book. As we teach, we've heard ourselves repeatedly say something of interest from a specific source, only to discover that when we looked for it, it was nowhere to be found in that book. The book had served its purpose. It stimulated our own creativity and our association to new knowledge. If you prefer to read this work in an uptime trance (so you can stay awake!), here's how to do it: sit comfortably (i.e., don't lie down), holding the book slightly farther away from your body than you do customarily and at approximately a forty-five degree angle. Read the pages more rapidly than usual, using your finger to skim them if necessary. To stay in an uptime trance, you need to dissociate from the material—a rapid read, with the book held at a slight distance, will make this possible.

So . . . . . . get ready . . . . . . settle back . . . . . . relax . . . . . . and just enjoy . . . . . . engaging in one of the finest examples of the wonders of your unconscious mind: reading. You may want to begin clarifying why reading this book is important to you, so by the time you reach Chapter One, you'll know. If there are passages where your conscious mind is not fully understanding something, we suggest that you keep on reading so that you discover the overall meaning and intent of the passage. After reading an enjoyable amount, allow a few hours or even a full night's sleep before you begin consciously reviewing and recalling the information that you read.

As you prepare to read the text, it may be useful for you to consider that your unconscious mind can *easily record all of the information in this book*. It *already* knows what is truly meaningful to you about reading this book and it knows why you want to read it. (It knew that when it motivated you to pick it up!) For us, one of the most exciting aspects about reading a book like this is wondering how the information, techniques, and learnings will surface over time and in what way. Part of our hope for you, as you read this book, is that you *begin to read in a whole new way*. Don't expect to know everything right away. Give your unconscious mind time to organize the information so that it is truly meaningful to you. Enjoy the process of not understanding everything. Look forward to being surprised at what you've learned and how it will be manifested in your work and in your life . . . . . . and in the meantime . . . . . . **remember** what Dr. Erickson would have said:

"You can pretend anything and master it."

TRAINING TRANCES

Chapter 1

Two Minds Defining Trances

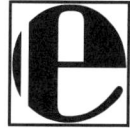

Editor's Notes: Chapters One and Two represent the foundation of this training. In Chapter One, the trainers present didactic information interspersed with hypnotic language. (The hypnotic language is italicized in the text for the ease of the reader.) The intention throughout this chapter is to pace and lead the group into trance without doing an overt trance induction. The trainers are calibrating to the development of trance and group rapport.

The left-brain information in this chapter represents the trainers' model of understanding which will be the basis of the training. The nature of the conscious and unconscious minds is discussed along with trance and hypnosis. Erickson's definition of the hypnotic state is included. This information is presented for at least two reasons. The first is for the value of the information itself. The second reason is to expand upon the participants' knowledge base so they can easily "step into" the therapeutic models being discussed. The trainers unfold this information as they calibrate to the audience's participation in the frames and presuppositions which the trainers are setting.

Since one of the major purposes of this chapter is preframing, no overt inductions, demonstrations, or exercises are included. This chapter ends with a brief question-and-answer segment.

We want to formally welcome you to *Training Trances,* a training in trance. This book is based upon information which we've synthesized from our knowledge of Neuro-Linguistic Programming and the work of Dr. Milton H. Erickson. Although there are techniques in this book which one can find elsewhere, our experience has taught us that it is the spirit and the personality of the practitioner which brings the techniques to life. Each person brings their own unique understanding to an approach or a set of techniques. What follows is ours. So hopefully you'll have an opportunity to *experience trance* in a whole new way by the end of the first reading if not sooner . . . not that *we're going to begin making suggestions* just yet, because it's more important at this point that you determine what it is that you want to accomplish by reading this book. We guarantee that your unconscious mind will take you only as far as you direct it, so take some time and *fully consider* this before you continue reading. We're glad you decided to *take the trance!*

Conscious-Unconscious Processing Trances

The first construct which merits discussion is that of the conscious and the unconscious mind. It's the basis of most methods of psychotherapy and hypnotherapy, and what is meant by these two terms is often, shall we say, diverse. When we talk about the conscious mind, we are referring to our present or current awareness. The amount of information we can hold in consciousness is limited: seven plus or minus two chunks of information.[1] If we're under stress, the "magic" number seven can be considerably diminished. Relative to the total amount of information that our nervous system receives, our conscious awareness is a thin thread. If the conscious mind is limited to that information to which we are attending, then the boundaries between the conscious and unconscious minds must be quite fluid to account for immediate shifts in awareness.

For example, think of the conscious mind as a narrowly focused band of awareness which can be directed on whatever we think is presently important. It's like a beam of light from a flashlight that can be directed through a large, darkened room. As we change the direction of the beam, different parts of the room can be see—parts that had always been there, but had previously gone unnoticed. Sometimes we may forget about the rest of the room, remaining narrowly focused on only what is lit and thinking that is all there is. When we think about who we are, we necessarily engage in conscious processing. Concluding we are only who we think we are is mistaking the lighted portion of the room for the entire room. No matter how we think of ourselves, we are more than that.

If your conscious mind represents your current awareness, then *your unconscious mind represents everything else.* However, simply applying the term "mind" to these complex processes causes an interesting phenomenon to occur. "Mind" is a nominalization, indicating that a fluid system of human sensory awareness has been turned from a process into something static, "a mind." As soon as this conversion to a nominalization occurs, we slip into the land of obvious metaphor, and from our point of view this is still a useful metaphor. The terms "conscious" and "unconscious" minds really refer to the *"functions"* of the (one) mind. Therefore what is commonly referred to as the conscious and unconscious minds are the functions which we associate with them. For our purposes, and apparently Dr. Erickson's purposes, this metaphor, while nominalizing complex processes, does have utility—more than you could know, consciously. Depending upon which expert you use as a reference, your nervous system may be receiving up to two million bits of information per second.[2] This information is almost completely outside of your conscious awareness. In addition to this, everything you've ever seen, heard, felt, smelled, tasted, and said to yourself, is recorded in some way in your unconscious mind.[3] Erickson referred to it as "the storehouse" of all your memories, beliefs, identities, values, and other filters which delete, distort, and generalize the information you receive. It's also the storehouse for your autonomic functioning.[4] Your so-called "autonomic nervous system" would generally fall within the aegis of your unconscious mind. It contains all of your habitual patterns (anything that you do automatically). This includes sensation and perception, emotional responses, respiration, digestion, and on a micro level, the biochemical functioning of all of the above, as well as the endocrine and immune systems.[5]

Based upon this, we believe the body is part of the unconscious mind and ultimately part of "Mind." Pribram's holographic model of memory suggests that every part of the body has within it the memory of the whole.[6] Intelligence abounds. Unconscious information is continually reverberating throughout the body. The current tidal wave of research on neuropeptides is pointing in this direction, to the extent that now even the term "neuropeptide" has become something of a misnomer! These little molecular messengers originally thought to be located only in the brain are now found throughout the entire body.[7] *Everything in the body is communicating with everything else and it's all happening unconsciously. No matter what you think you are, you are more than that.*

Each mind and its related functions have inherent value in and of themselves, yet the two also combine in a mutually interdependent, co-existing system. The findings of Benjamin Libet, an innovative brain researcher, suggest that conscious will does not initiate an act, but rather selects and controls the outcome.[8] Other research indicates that the conscious mind, while limited in capacity, excels in context sensitivity, internal consistency, and serial processing. The unconscious mind is capable of engaging in diverse and highly specialized tasks which may, at times, even be contradictory to one another.[9]

An analogy which clarifies this relationship is one of the Captain and the Ship. The conscious mind is the Captain. Its primary responsibility is to set the course or direction—someone needs to know where the ship is headed. The unconscious is both the crew and the ship. The primary responsibility of the unconscious is to carry out the Captain's orders; it is the "doer." The Captain delegates all of the tasks to the crew for them to carry out; the Captain also checks the ship (the body) to make sure it's strong and sturdy. What often happens with an overactive conscious mind is, like a harried Captain, it thinks it must do every job itself rather than trusting the unconscious mind and letting it do the job for which it was designed. If the crew need the Captain's attention, they can call the Captain: otherwise a good Captain will trust the crew members to do their jobs. When there is mutual respect and understanding of their separate functions, they multiply their strengths and insure smooth sailing.

A "daily life" example of this happened recently. I was running late and looked at my watch as I walked into a meeting. My watch read 9:05 a.m. My conscious mind said, "I want to leave here by 9:30 a.m." I entered the meeting and forgot what time it was because I trusted my unconscious mind to do its job. I left the meeting and noted, as I waited to cross the street, that it was exactly 9:30 a.m.! That's a clear example of how the conscious mind acts as the "director" and the unconscious as the "doer."

Erickson's Unconscious Development

Erickson didn't necessarily begin his career viewing the unconscious as we have described above. When he began his training, he was in the generation which was still influenced by the work of Sigmund Freud. Freud's view of the unconscious mind was largely that it was an area where there were repressed negative emotions, deep-seated urges, and rampant sexual fantasies. Should we say a less-than-healthy view of the unconscious mind? Erickson was influenced initially by Freudian theory. It was primarily through his own clinical experience and his keen powers of observation that he synthesized a more practical and holistic view of the unconscious mind. His theory of the unconscious mind grew and developed over sixty years of experience in reportedly working with as many as 30,000 clients.[10]

Early in his career Erickson began to question the role of the unconscious mind, its real function, and how to best describe it. He developed the position that the unconscious is simultaneously a storehouse of all that is helpful and beneficial, as well as a storehouse of emotions, habits, and patterns which may no longer serve the individual.

As we said earlier, many of us mistake who we consciously think we are for the totality of who we are. We are much more than we think we are! Erickson believed that utilizing only the conscious mind was a limited view of one's resources and of the world itself. Only by getting in touch with the information in the storehouse could we really make the best decisions for ourselves. That's why he said it's so important to *"trust your unconscious mind."*

Trusting Your Unconscious . . . Processing

Interestingly, we may not really have any choice on a neurological level but to trust our unconscious minds. In 1979, Benjamin Libet published a landmark paper on what he called "subjective referral."[11] In a series of ingenious experiments he demonstrated that conscious awareness occurs only about a half-second (500 milliseconds) after the time a stimulus is introduced. This makes sense, in that it takes time to develop the electrical activity which eventually results in conscious awareness. Here's the interesting twist. Even though a half-second elapses from the time a stimulus is introduced to the time we are conscious of it, it appears to us as if no delay in awareness has occurred and we are accurate at identifying the time and the stimulus. We make a subjective referral back in time based on our unconscious kinesthetic memory of the initial stimulus. What this means is we probably *do everything unconsciously first*. So the time-honored definition of conscious awareness being "that to which we are currently aware" is really a projection of our unconscious mind! The moral of the story: trust your unconscious mind. You'll *produce alignment and harmony in yourself* when you do.

An advantage to working with the unconscious mind and relying on it is that it's able to process things in a simultaneous way which the conscious mind is unable to do. The conscious mind thinks in a sequential, linear way, whereas the *unconscious mind is able to do almost an infinite number of things independently of the conscious mind*. For example, you don't have to think about breathing in order for respiration to occur. Now, you can put your consciousness on that, but you don't have to be paying attention to your breathing right now in order for your unconscious mind to allow you to breathe in exactly the way in which you need.

This simultaneous and independent functioning of your unconscious mind includes more than just the autonomic, regulatory activities which we need to physically stay alive. There is an ever-growing body of evidence supporting the pervasive nature of unconscious learning.[12] As early as the 1960s,[13] studies supported the idea of latent learning; that we can *learn things purely unconsciously and later retrieve the information*.

Perhaps equally significant are the many studies which suggest that information learned unconsciously can be stored in long-term memory, having the potential for long term influence of behavior without any conscious mediation.[14] Brain researchers have proposed what they call the Internal Processing Algorithm (IPA) which is the strategy used to acquire information unconsciously.[15] It's the way we decide what we will *learn* (not just record) *unconsciously* and what we won't. (There is ample evidence of this in our lives: remembering bits of a conversation someone else was having at a party while we were engaged in a conversation of our own; remembering lyrics of a song we heard on the radio while driving even though we didn't think we were paying attention to the radio; or hearing an alarm clock while sleeping and incorporating it into a dream.) This was one of Erickson's greatest insights: that these two minds can and do operate independently from one another while creating a synergistic effect. (He recognized this well before researchers documented it in the laboratory.) This last notion of parallel processing opens many possibilities in terms of formulating a dynamic and flexible model of the world which will be discussed more fully in later sections.

The other thing we ought to talk about is ..... *Trance* .... *now!* ......

Defining Trances

What is hypnosis? It's one of those things like aspirin: a lot of people have used it but don't have a clue as to why or how it works. It's a slippery subject to define. Physicists have questioned, "What is light?" and therapists have questioned, "What is hypnosis?"

Erickson's concept of hypnosis was much broader than some of his contemporaries because he believed that it was something which was naturally occurring. It was a part of everyday life and could be found anywhere: in elevators, in libraries, in cars, in movie theaters, in lovers' eyes, in dreams, and so on. Our view is that he thought of hypnosis this way not only as a result of his own autohypnotic experiences, but also because having a broader definition was pragmatic. Recognizing hypnosis as an everyday phenomenon makes it far more accessible to the everyday person.

In fact, toward the latter part of his career, he didn't use the word "hypnosis" as much as the word "trance." Nobody knows exactly why that is. Andre Weitzenhoffer, a colleague of Erickson, hypothesized that Erickson very much wanted people to accept hypnosis[16] and for a good bit of his career Erickson was considered to be a maverick. Hypnosis, itself, had a similar reputation of being unusual and far-fetched. Therefore, one of the things Erickson wanted to do was to restore credibility to the field of Hypnosis. One of the possible explanations for his use of the word "trance" was that hypnosis had certain connotations which he didn't want people to associate with his work. So he started calling it trance, which seemed to be a more acceptable, generic term. He used those two words, as best we can tell, interchangeably. Therefore, we may talk about trance or about hypnosis, and for our purposes, we're talking about the same thing.

Trance Is A State You Live In

Think of hypnosis or trance as a state of being, an altered state of awareness. An altered state is by definition any state that's different in some way from the normal, waking state.[17] Hypnosis is biologically similar to the hypnogogic state (the transition from waking to sleeping), the hypnopompic state (the transition from sleeping to waking), and the dream state. There is a considerable body of research indicating strong similarities between hypnosis and dreaming in EEG activity, cortical and subcortical stimulation, and neurotransmitter activity.[18] In fact, the underlying mechanism for dreaming (rapid eye movement sleep) continues to operate through the entire waking state represented as ultradian cycles.[19] We're always cycling through biological rhythms that make trance a naturally occurring state.

Ernest Rossi believes that the everyday trance state to which Erickson often referred is a direct result of these ultradian rhythms.[20] This is probably the most scientifically compelling basis for believing that everyone can enter trance. Trance, at least in part, is a state driven by a set of predictable biological mechanisms. Rossi noted that particularly in his later years, Erickson would wait until he noticed the patient "quieting down."[21] Rather than having to do lengthy ritualistic inductions, many times it was just a matter of catching the client when they were in one of these states. (We'll return to this idea when we discuss utilization and trance induction.)

When we talk about hypnosis in a therapeutic sense, we're generally talking about it as an inner-directed state. As the person's awareness becomes more and more focused upon their internal thoughts, processes, or sensations, they are eliciting the trance state within themselves. As Spiegel puts it, "[It's] a state of attentive, receptive focal concentration with a sense of parallel awareness...."[22]

Erickson On Trance

Erickson's definition explains why using trance is important and also addresses the question of when and why you would use it. Someone once asked, "Dr. Erickson, why do you use hypnosis, and what is hypnosis?" Erickson replied (we're paraphrasing here), *"The hypnotic state is a state in which the client pays attention to what is really, immediately important, and disregards information that isn't immediately important. In an hypnotic state, you may not be aware of your right foot, you may not be aware of your right arm, or that you're wearing a watch. You can just forget about that. You can forget about your left arm, you can forget about what you had for breakfast. You can forget about anything that is up here on the board while you're listening to what I'm saying. What's important about the hypnotic trance is that you're capable of paying attention to what is immediately important so that you can access memories and resources that you have long since forgotten.*"[23] His whole idea was that whenever he wanted someone to pay attention . . . . he'd use trance or hypnotic techniques.

You may be familiar with "ordeals" in Ericksonian work where he would task a client to go out and weed the rose garden or something like that for some therapeutic reason. Some of the tasks were quite novel, to say the least. Other clinicians would wonder how he could motivate his clients to do this. He could get them to do unusual tasks because he used the trance state to do these things. Anytime he had something he thought was important for the client to understand, he would use trance. Erickson used trance as an amplifier of communication. Trance makes it possible for us to delete massive amounts of information that are not salient so we can magnify and focus on relevant material and consider it in new ways. Hypnosis amplifies and magnifies the important communication which we want to trans . . . mit to the other person!

Erickson frequently even used trance when he made presentations to associations or formal committee meetings! Most participants probably weren't consciously aware of what he was doing. He'd speak to them in his low, gravelly "trance voice" and he might go on for hours. Most of the participants would be in trance and reportedly often had amnesia for the content, but on a deeper level they understood something important was occurring.

In trance, they would no longer pay attention to the unimportant parts, they'd pay attention to the important things because trance speaks to the unconscious part of the mind. If you want to talk to someone, you can speak to their conscious mind (seven plus or minus two chunks of awareness) or to their unconscious, which is everything else in their experience.

Erickson wanted to speak to the unconscious, because he knew the conscious mind wasn't going to make important decisions. He understood that he had to utilize trance to access the broad range of their experience. The trance would direct their attention by focusing it. He narrowed their attention to a single laser beam of concentration. As he created this narrowly focused trance, he layered in his suggestions and the information which he wanted them to understand. He'd work with the unconscious because it was the only part of the individual that was going to make those choices anyhow. It's legendary that Erickson used trance or hypnotic techniques for everything he did—talking to his kids, working with his clients, giving seminars, even talking to the gardener!

He might say, "Whenever I am talking to you, I want your unconscious to fully consider, fully consider what's being said. Not that you're necessarily going to accept it, but that you will fully *consider it at a deeper level.*" So that's what he was really looking for when he was working with people. He would be using trance most of the time, although there may not have been an obvious, formal kind of trance. He used hypnotic principles to create a naturalistic trance when observers were looking for formal inductions.

Richard Bandler, who has modeled some of Erickson's approaches, also suggests that hypnosis is an amplifier of experience.[24] Richard's view, as we understand it, is that any NLP technique will often create trance by presupposition, i.e. as the client's attention focuses narrowly on the technique she/he goes into trance. Richard's addition to this is if you take an NLP technique and put it inside of trance, you amplify the effects of that particular technique and, therefore, the internal experience of the listener.

Another reason why hypnosis is useful is because it suspends and bypasses normal, conscious limitations.[25] "Helping the patient get out of his own way," is how Erickson described it.[26] As clients *fully consider what's being said* with their unconscious mind, they're no longer just considering it with their normal conscious mindsets. They are then in a state of suspended awareness. Oftentimes people will recognize that they have a problem or behavior which they want to change and they will try to change it consciously. They'll "try" to remember "not" to do it again; sooner or later, they are caught off guard and the old behavior occurs automatically. Using a purely conscious approach with repetitive issues, which are the domain of the unconscious mind, is like saying apples and oranges are the same because they are fruit. Change must occur in the domain where the problem exists. The solution ought to be as automatic as the problem once was. That's what produces elegant change.

Sensory Awareness Rings True

To work in an elegant fashion with the client's unconscious mind, Erickson trained himself to make very acute observations about which nonverbals accompanied the verbal message. If he noticed an incongruity in their communication, he might have asked himself, "What part of their physiology matches their words (perhaps the conscious mind) and what part matches their unconscious response (perhaps their body)?" He understood how important it is to calibrate to unconscious responses. If you don't *remember everything that's been taught in this training,* then remember this: what made Erickson famous, as well as effective as a healer, wasn't his technique. The techniques he utilized are what you're always taught, but it wasn't his technique that made him the genius he was. It was his power of observation, his calibration skills, and his ability to *make very, very fine sensory distinctions,* which made him so effective in assisting others to change their lives.

If a therapist is not trained to make fine distinctions, she/he may be referred to as a technician who operates in a vacuum of their own hallucinations.

The therapist's success ratio may be relatively low because they're imposing a preset pattern without calibrating to the individual's unconscious responses. A number of scientific studies devoted to hypnosis demonstrated this limitation. In one instance, a clinician in a white lab coat read a script to a subject. After doing this, the researchers discovered only twenty percent of the subjects were susceptible to trance. What they didn't realize was the twenty percent who were susceptible to trance were also naturally somnambulistic.[27] "Coincidentally" somnambulism comprises twenty percent of the population.[28] One out of five people will naturally access trance regardless of the protocol used. If clinicians would customize what they do to suit participants' preference for accessing trance, their success ratio would improve significantly. Erickson knew how to assist almost everyone with going into a trance because he based his trance induction on his observation of the client and their individual needs.

Erickson was an expert at knowing when he had a person's unconscious attention. There's a great story of a woman who was participating in a hypnosis demonstration with Erickson in Philadelphia.[29] She had been his student in the past. Erickson was working with her to demonstrate certain hypnotic phenomena, and as the interview progressed a light trance was occurring but without any display of the intended hypnotic phenomena. So, here was the master, Erickson, with Andre Weitzenhoffer, Jay Haley, and a number of other people observing, and the demonstration was not going the way they had planned.

Erickson finally sat back and realized that this woman did not have on her engagement ring, nor did she have on a wedding ring. No one said a word to him about this, and she never said a word. When he had seen her the year before, she had an engagement ring on her finger. So Erickson took a piece of paper and rolled it up, and began to go over his ring finger with the paper. He didn't say anything to her as he dropped the paper on the floor; he didn't talk about this at all; he just did this totally unconsciously, and then he said something along the lines of, ".... and now moving right along ...." Then he picked up where he left off, and she went into a deep trance and exhibited the hypnotic phenomena which he wanted to demonstrate.

The message he gave her unconscious mind was, "I know about this." When he went over the ring finger with the paper, he called attention to his finger, and then he threw the paper onto the floor as if he was done with it. When they interviewed him later, he said he calibrated to her unconscious mind's refusal to enter trance as an expression of fear. If she allowed herself to go into trance, she thought it may be exposed that she didn't go through with the engagement or the marriage. She was afraid this issue was going to be exposed in front of all these people. Erickson had to reassure her somehow in that moment, and that's how he chose to communicate directly with her unconscious. To me, that was a brilliant piece of work. That's what has inspired me to make fine distinctions with my clients so that I respect their unconscious intentions. Erickson's elegance demonstrates the value of calibration and the utilization of hypnotic principles.

This is why he remarked (and others have concurred) that for each client, he did therapy differently. He observed the idiosyncratic details of each client's life and experience and used this individualized information to leverage change. Much of what he did was exclusive to that particular individual. There were, of course, some commonalities from one client to the next, but he would only make generalizations after he had verified them over a period of time. His most effective means of verification was to go into trance himself so he could *pay very close attention* to people.

Discussion

DON: How would you handle it if you had a client who had a previous hypnosis session and concluded from it that hypnosis doesn't work?

Here's a helpful distinction to mention when you're defining hypnosis to a client or audience. First, as we mentioned, hypnosis is a state, not a technique. Hypnosis is an altered state of awareness. We have, however, often used the word "hypnosis" to describe a technique, so when we say, "I'm doing hypnosis with my client," or "I'm using hypnosis with my client," the meaning can be misleading. We ought to more properly say, "I'm assisting my client in accessing (the state of) hypnosis."

If you answer the question or respond to the client by agreeing, "Hypnosis doesn't work," or something like that, you've bought into their model of the world. How's that possible? Think of it this way. If someone says, "Hypnosis doesn't work," you might want to say something like, "That's right, I want you to consider that hypnosis doesn't work in the same way that confidence doesn't work, or security doesn't work, or enthusiasm doesn't work, or relaxation doesn't work...." The only way a particular state wouldn't work is if it's not appropriate to the context. Confidence isn't a technique, it's a state in the same way hypnosis is a state.

DOT: I have a patient who's had years of hypnotherapy, so she can get herself immediately into a trance, and at times I have to fight not going into the trance with her.

You have to fight going into a trance?

DOT: Well, I don't know whether I should be fighting it or going into it. That was my question.

Think of it this way: if you want to be in rapport with her, and since rapport is the basis of any kind of effective human interaction, then it would probably be worthwhile to be in trance. However, the <u>type</u> of trance that you're in is a different trance than the client's. She's probably in a downtime, or inside trance, which is what we're going to talk about. Her attention is inward—she's accessing possibilities, associations, and memories. Your trance, which you're going to have an experience of in the first exercise as a hypnotherapist, is to be in an uptime, or outside trance. An uptime trance is a heightened state of external, sensory awareness.

DOT: I'm aware of that, and it frees me up to just go with the right kinds of questions, and I don't have to think about what I'm going to ask her.

Right.

DOT: At times it feels I have a sense that I could go so far into my trance that I wouldn't be able to be in control of the session.

Has that ever happened?

DOT: No.

And I wonder what part of your mind has the sense that you could go too far with that trance?

DOT: I don't trust my unconscious mind . . . .

Your conscious and unconscious minds are not working together so *you can trust yourself.*

DOT At times I just want to go with her.

As you continue in this training, we'd like you to enjoy just going with trance here, because it's safe to experience the trance state <u>as the hypnotherapist</u>. Just let yourself *be totally comfortable* going to the most appropriate depth of trance for you to be an excellent hypnotherapist and see how it feels. Then you can decide for yourself if it's an effective way to do therapy. Actually, most people don't realize the best way to prevent burnout is by utilizing trance in <u>themselves</u> as they do therapy.

MEREDITH:
    I've noticed that I'm great at going into trance in stores!

That's good. As long as you remember to get the change, it doesn't matter if you forget that you're in a trance. "Store" trance. I always thought you should store trance as long as you take the change with you. Either way is perfect.

So we have *trance*, we have *hypnosis*, we have the conscious and *you're unconscious*, and you are already to . . . . *learn more!* SO . . . . . .

Chapter 2

What Do Driving And Garages Have To Do With Intention And Trance?

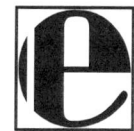

Editor's Note: Chapter Two expands upon the information included in the first chapter. The trainers discuss the nature of suggestion and define direct and indirect suggestion. The highlight and centerpiece of this chapter is a superb double induction, aptly entitled "Driving Trances." A major induction such as this sets up the entire training by communicating certain information and presuppositions directly to the unconscious mind. While depotentiating the conscious minds of the audience, it is also a demonstration of group trance. The longer paragraphs of the induction generally represent just one trainer speaking in a hypnotic voice. The "one-liners" represent the trainers' hypnotic language, which sometimes occurred simultaneously, and at other times sequentially. The challenge to the reader is to hear the induction while reading it.

"Driving Trances" also becomes the setup for the first exercise. While still in trance (albeit a lighter one) the participants move into the "That's Right" exercise. Questions from the audience follow as the chapter ends with a discussion of the importance of holding positive internal representations.

Question to the reader: Several "loops" (incomplete pieces of information or unanswered questions) are opened in this chapter. How many are there?

Does Ericksonian Hypnotherapy Really Exist?

One of the things that Dr. Erickson was famous for, particularly during the latter part of his career, was telling stories and metaphors. We hope that all of you are inspired to go back and read his original publications. Many of his case studies read like novels and are as entertaining as they are therapeutic. After reading his work and listening to his therapies, an inescapable irony emerges: **Erickson didn't do Ericksonian Hypnotherapy. Erickson did what he needed to do based upon what he was observing.** His students codified what he did and called it Ericksonian Hypnotherapy, but <u>he</u> didn't do Ericksonian Hypnotherapy.

Many people don't realize that much of what Erickson did evolved from his early exposure to traditional, authoritarian hypnosis. His first formal training in hypnosis was in a seminar with Clark Hull. Hull, a renowned researcher in hypnosis at that time, subscribed to a standardized approach for inducing trance.[1] Erickson's use of indirection as a therapeutic method occurred in part as a reaction to this traditional, standardized approach, where the same induction was used for each person.[2] His personal experiences with self-hypnosis, his clinical research, and ideas stimulated by theoreticians of his era such as Boris Sidis, George Estabrooks, and Andre Weitzenhoffer all contributed to his unique style of hypnosis. Our observation is that when Erickson realized the traditional, direct approach was only going to reach a limited population, he began to experiment with indirect suggestion. Later in Erickson's career, after he had used the indirect approach for some time, he began concentrating very heavily on the use of stories and therapeutic metaphors to accomplish his goals. At this stage of his career, having built such a huge reference base which directed his exceptional powers of observation, he dispensed with a lot of the obvious ritual which many recognized as "hypnotism."

Today, when we're talking about Ericksonian approaches or techniques, we're talking about a more <u>permissive</u> <u>approach</u> to working with a person, as opposed to an authoritarian approach where we would say, "You will go into a trance." We wouldn't do that. What's the point of saying, *"Your eyes are getting heavier . . . . your eyes are blinking . . . . your eyes keep blinking . . . . your eyes are getting heavier . . . . and heavier . . . . . you're listening to what I'm saying . . . . you hear only what I'm saying . . . . you feel your eyes getting heavy and you're starting to get sleepier . . . . you notice the changes . . . . you want to sleep . . . . . your eyes close and you go into a deep sleep, sleep . . . . just sleep."* That's going to work easily and effectively for only a small group of people. Generally speaking, this will be one out of five people.[3]

If we were using an indirect, permissive approach, we would say, *"You <u>can</u> go into a trance if you'd like, and I wonder how you'd like to do that? Maybe you'd just like to relax in the chair where you are sitting . . . . or maybe there's something else that you could think about that would relax you even more . . . . in any event . . . you can just go on listening and paying attention to what I'm saying in any way that you wish."* That's much more permissive and indirect and relies on presupposition, as opposed to stating directly what the subject is to do.

In traditional hypnosis, the hypnotist told the subject what to do and expected them to do it. Erickson's position was if we tell someone what to do, and they don't do it, we ought to do something else instead. Erickson believed that we need to tailor the approach for eliciting trance to the particular individual with whom we are working. Therefore, we base what we say and do on what we observe our client doing. We calibrate to—their *head nods,* their *breathing,* their *smile,* how they're *sitting in their chair,* their increasing *relaxation* . . . . . . that's Ericksonian suggestion. We tailor it to the individual person rather than imposing a set protocol upon them. The Ericksonian approach goes with the flow; and mirrors and matches the individual on all levels. By contrast, traditional hypnotists often used scripts which they delivered in a monotone voice, perhaps repeating the same thing over and over until the subject became so bored that they'd go into a trance.

Our view is that a necessary and sufficient condition for the hypnotic relationship is symmetry, often referred to as rapport. Mirroring and matching are two ways of creating symmetry in the relationship. A recent study highlighted this point. Researchers measured physiological changes in the respiration, GSR, EEG, cardiovascular, and muscle responses of both therapists and clients, and demonstrated that synchronization of these responses were "strongly" correlated with trance. Perhaps even more importantly, the researchers also observed that a lack of synchronization relative to these responses between the therapist and the client prevented the trance state from developing.[4] Synchronization is analogous to rapport. Erickson's genius was that he recognized that many people were incongruent about going into trance and he learned how to establish rapport with them so they could "synch up."

As we consider it now, the subjects who were considered "highly susceptible" or "highly suggestible" by traditional standards (the one in five) were probably more congruent about going into a trance. This congruency would then lead to rapport and the occurrence of trance. Therefore, direct requests could be made with these subjects and they would follow them. But what about the other eighty percent who were labelled "average" or even "refractory?" In these latter cases, there was no symmetry in the overall relationship between the hypnotist and the subject. They didn't "synch up" with one another so trance never resulted. Erickson realized that to the extent the hypnotist could mirror or pace the incongruencies of the subject, the overall relationship between them would become symmetrical and would dramatically increase the likelihood of trance. This was one of Erickson's most valuable contributions to the field of hypnosis.

InDirect Suggestion: What Are You Noticing?

There's another principle which we think is very useful and which isn't commonly discussed in Hypnosis. We first found it in the book, *Psychology of Suggestion,* by Boris Sidis, which was published in 1898. He was one of the first writers to discuss the difference between direct and indirect suggestion.[5] Initially, in Ericksonian work as done by the neo-Ericksonians, the idea was to become as indirect as possible whenever you had the opportunity. Erickson was even quoted, more or less, as saying the same thing.[6] His reason for taking the position that indirect suggestion was preferable was probably that many of his clients had overactive conscious minds. The clients who had not succeeded with other hypnotherapists or therapists usually fell into this category, and that's often whom Erickson had as clients. Using indirect language depotentiates the conscious mind, i.e. gets it out of the way.[7]

Based upon this, a number of the Ericksonians advocate indirect suggestion almost exclusively. Many times in their therapies, they utilize indirect methods for not only the trance induction but also for the changework. There's only one problem. When the client is in a deeper hypnotic state, the conscious mind isn't there and the unconscious mind is. Indirect suggestions are basically useful for getting the conscious mind out of the way. Once the client is in trance, the unconscious mind comes to the forefront while the conscious mind recedes. The unconscious mind then operates on the principle of literalism. When a person is deeply in trance, the hypnotherapist needs to be as specific as possible. That's really important!

The graph on the following page shows that one variable would be the type of suggestions (direct to indirect) and the other variable would be the depth of trance (waking to somnambulism).

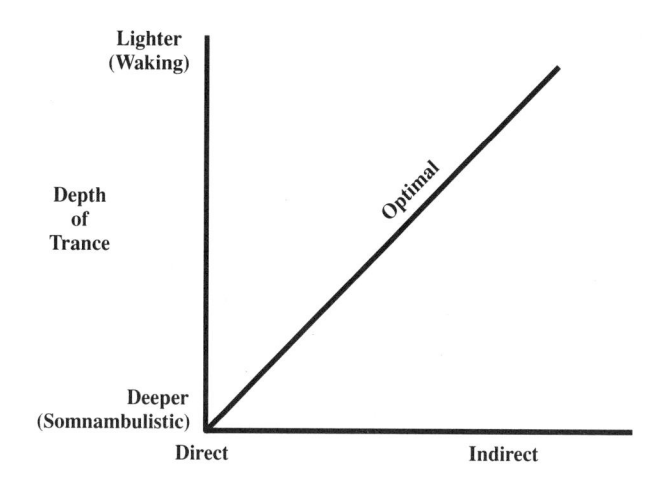

[Figure: A graph with "Depth of Trance" on the y-axis (ranging from "Lighter (Waking)" at top to "Deeper (Somnambulistic)" at bottom) and "Relative Directness of Suggestions" on the x-axis (from "Direct" to "Indirect"). A diagonal line labeled "Optimal" extends from lower-left to upper-right.]

Figure 2.1 *The lighter the trance and closer to normal waking functioning, the more indirect "you <u>can</u> become." The deeper the trance, the more direct "you <u>will</u> become."*

There is a relationship between the type of suggestion made and the depth of trance. Indirect suggestion is best utilized when the person is in a waking trance[8] or earlier in the trance induction. As the client goes deeper and deeper into trance, the more direct the suggestions become.[9] Erickson used both direct and indirect suggestion. In his transcripts, he becomes more direct as trance develops. At certain points, he actually tells people exactly what he wants them to do. The significance of this will become clearer as we go on. What's important to remember is once a person's in a deep trance, that's when their unconscious mind will respond best to direct suggestion.

Let's take a moment and define what we mean by direct and indirect suggestion. With "indirect" suggestion, choices are provided. The language allows choice and possibility. With "direct" suggestion, one statement regarding a behavior, belief, or value that the person is to do is presented, with the expectation of a direct response which is the actualization of the particular behavior. In direct suggestion, the language is often stated as, "You will, you shall, you are." It often uses direct commands. Indirect suggestion provides more possibility, by leaving choice open to the unconscious mind to do whatever it wants. If you're interested in the language patterns of indirect suggestion, please see the Milton Model in the Appendix.

For example, a standard indirect suggestion which we use is: "I don't know how you'll integrate your new learnings tonight while you sleep because we all dream . . . Some of you might have wild dreams, boring dreams, crazy dreams . . . Some of you might have dreams with casts of thousands or dreams with casts of a few . . . some of you may even think you've had no dreams at all and let that be a sign that the learnings are occurring!" That's indirect suggestion because the listener is choosing which response to have in their dreams. They pick the response from selections which all presuppose the same thing: *you'll have dreams of integration.*

It's appropriate in the earlier phases of trance that clients have multiple choices, so they feel they're in control. Once they are in a deep trance, we believe their unconscious responds to requests similarly to how a child of six or seven years old would respond. In a medium to deep trance, their unconscious mind will respond very literally to the suggestions presented (just as a young child would before their conscious mind develops). When they are in a medium to deep trance you want to make direct suggestions. This is a good time for you to directly suggest whatever the outcome of the session is and calibrate to their responses. With direct suggestion, your expectation is they will follow through with one response which was provided in the suggestion.

The type of the suggestion used (direct or indirect) may also determine the way it is carried out. Direct suggestion tends to create a full and <u>complete realization</u> of the suggestion, or an "immediate" response. What Sidis referred to as a "mediate" response is an activation or an actualization of <u>associations</u> to the suggestion, via contiguity of time and space or similarity and contrast.[10] Rather than suggesting something directly, associations are created. Different associations are activated within the unconscious, and the client carries out the suggestion based upon the associations they make during trance.

Here's an easy way to check which form of suggestion clients will respond to best. This is a quick and easy diagnostic tool. I'll use an extreme example to illustrate this point. Right now I want you to make your mouth water. Your mouth will water . . . make your mouth water . . . your mouth is watering . . . your mouth is watering . . . your mouth is watering. How many of you notice that your mouth starts to water? That's a very direct suggestion.

Now, a more indirect suggestion would be something like this: all of you know what it's like to hold a lemon in your hand? And what it's like when you bring that lemon up to your mouth and take a big bite from it? How many of you got a stronger response with that?

The idea in the first one is we told you your mouth would water. The second one is an attempt at opening up or activating neural networks by making associations. One's direct and the other's more indirect. The optimal way to work is to utilize both. If you create associations and the person's mouth begins to water, then you say, "Your mouth will water" and it will deepen the level of rapport in the hypnotic relationship.

What Do Driving And Garages Have To Do With Intention And Trance?

Interestingly enough, the latest research on suggestion indicates that both direct and indirect suggestion are effective and that neither is more potent than the other.[11] Erickson used whichever method was required based on the individual's hypnotic ability within that particular context.[12] The issue of importance is not which one works best, but who actually increases the effectiveness of the suggestion which is provided. At present, two keys to increased effectiveness include how the suggestions are presented[13] and the context in which they occur.[14] Is there a relationship of rapport and positive expectation (or intention) and are the suggestions delivered in a manner which paces the client's model of the world? If they are, then whether direct or indirect suggestion is used, the overall effectiveness of hypnosis is increased.

Speaking of effectiveness, do you recognize one of the greatest "trance mediums" for suggestion? The TV. Watch the advertisements and notice how suggestions are utilized on a larger scale. They often utilize indirect suggestion first, by creating associations, then at the end of the commercial, by firing off a direct suggestion. When Bill Clinton ran for the presidency, some of his ads began with old clips of John F. Kennedy and Martin Luther King. They created the associations with old footage (one even used John-John Kennedy at his father's funeral) which stirred up the viewers' emotions. Then they finished with a bold one-liner: "Vote for Clinton." They created associations which were indirect and which fixated attention (creating trance)—then they gave the direct suggestion to vote for Clinton. If the viewer accepted the associations because they were in alignment with their values, the "Vote for Clinton" message went right into their unconscious mind without resistance. That's a very powerful and elegant use of hypnotic principles in everyday life.

You may have already noticed from the above examples that all communication may be thought of as a form of suggestion. Even this last sentence was a . . . . suggestion. Trance is a naturally occurring phenomenon. Many times the most effective suggestions may go unnoticed, sometimes not.

As we mentioned earlier, in Erickson's later career he was using stories, anecdotes, and metaphors so frequently that some of the more traditional hypnotherapists wondered if he was even doing trance anymore! He seemed to be just sitting around talking to people. They may have even wondered if he was "losing it," because all he appeared to be doing was telling stories. He might tell stories for hours straight, and to the untrained ear, some seemed only marginally connected. People would leave and have amnesia about the stories which he told them. Some thought they had wasted their time hearing this man droning on and on. Interestingly, after they left, somehow their lives would change and, for some curious reason, they would start referring all their friends to him. Their unconscious minds understood that when he told a story, he was speaking directly to them.

A Story

From our research, it appears that Erickson moved up through the ranks of his profession very quickly—he began as an assistant resident and psychiatrist and then was promoted to full psychiatrist at Worcester State Hospital, which, at the time, was arguably one of the top research hospitals in the country. He later moved to Wayne County General Hospital in Eloise, Michigan. He practiced there for about fifteen years and remarried during that time.

Anyway, after being there for about fifteen years, Erickson had a problem. Some of you may know that, at age eighteen, he recovered successfully from a bout with polio. Depending upon whom you talk to, they say his problem was muscle cramps or allergies that may have been a residual effect from the polio.[15] So, since he had this problem, we wondered what it would have been like if he had sought some advice. We also wondered what it would have been like if he'd decided to seek assistance from a friend of his who was a lot like him . . . and another physician.

The physician interviewed Milton and said, "So Dr. Erickson, *why are you here?* What are you really here for? What is the problem that you are having?" Erickson thought about it for a minute and said, "I've got these allergies and this discomfort, and I'm really hoping that you can help me." The doctor looked at him and said, "Let's see what we can do."

He went over all the information, asking Milton some other questions and finally came up with his conclusion, and he said, "Milton, I do know what you want, and I know how *you can solve that problem that you have,* and you can, you know." Milton was listening. He continued, "Milton, *I'm willing to tell you what it is that you can do to resolve this on one condition.*"

Erickson thought about it and replied, "Okay, what is it?" The doctor said, *"Whatever I tell you to do, I want you to do it."* Erickson said, "Okay." The doctor said, "Milton, *you came here for a specific reason, you have a very specific thing that you want to get rid of,* and as far as I can tell, the only way that you're really going to be able to get rid of these allergies and arthritis from living in the climate and environment that you've been in, is you are going to need to . . . *change* . . . *states* of residence."

Milton just sat there with a blank look on his face and said, "What?" The doctor said, "That's right, Milton. If you're going to get what you really want, you're going to need to *change states* . . . of residence. The sooner the better."

Of course, different people would interpret what was just said in different ways. Some people, when told to change states of residence, would probably move, maybe from one state to the next one, like Minnesota . . .

What Do Driving And Garages Have To Do With Intention And Trance? 23

Double Induction

JOHN: ... If you were ambitious, you'd go all the way to North Dakota. But see, Milton was extremely ambitious. When somebody told him to change states of residence, he took it seriously. He took it *all the way* into the *deep* Southwest of the United States. We don't really know how he traveled to get there; he could have flown, or he could have driven.

JULIE: There are a lot of ways to get where you want to go to. I think he took the highway ...

JOHN: ... in our opinion the high ... way is the best way ...

JULIE: ... now those of you, who don't know it as the highway ...

JOHN: ... may know it as the ...

JULIE: ... freeway ...

JOHN: ... free ... way and that's just as good in our opinion ...

JULIE: ... in fact, for some of you either is better ...

JOHN: ... you can just take the interstate ...

JULIE: ... the inner ... state that runs through the United States ...

JOHN: ... to get to ...

JULIE: ... your state ...

JOHN: ... that you're headed toward. Now, I'm not really sure, which way did he go?

JULIE: ... I think Erickson took ... did you ever take a driving trance?

JOHN: ... driving trances are the ones with the most mobility ...

JULIE: ... driving trance, that's a moving experience ... a driving trance

JOHN: . . . something we all take for granted, too, because there was a time when you couldn't drive, and when you learned all those things that you had to put together at the same time. You had to be steering, you had to know just the right amount of pressure. When were you supposed to brake and when were you to accelerate?

JULIE: . . . even when you learned to drive, it was really driving you were doing . . . And when you've gone on a long trip and you've had a co-pilot or a navigator beside you, who's really been the person driving? Is it the person holding the steering wheel, or the person who knows where they are going? Sometimes the driver thinks he knows, but sometimes only the navigator knows for sure on the high . . . way how to get right where you're going . . . and Milton was going to the Deep . . . . Southwest.

JOHN: . . . even deeper . . .

JULIE: . . . all the way down . . .

JOHN: . . . down the inner state . . .

JULIE: . . . and only at your rate, because in this type of driving trance, you can drive eighty-five, and it's legal in this state. You can drive ninety-five. Some of you have already broken one hundred and are going quickly and more deeply into trance. It's just your trance, just your state . . .

JOHN: . . . who should tell you how fast to drive in your state?

JULIE: . . . others of you might want to slow down in your trance, because not everyone likes to drive, those people can just sit still and be driven, that's right. So we're not really sure how Erickson did get to Ari-zona . . .

JOHN: . . . one thing we do know is that after you've been in a driving trance for this long, certainly your unconscious drives the car. And one good thing about all unconscious drivers is they all know how to *signal* their *intentions* whenever they're about to change directions . . .

JULIE: . . . and they don't do that until they **see the proper signs,** the signs that let you know it's time to **signal** your **intentions before you change** . . . . lanes . . .

JOHN: . . . before you make the next turn . . .

JULIE: . . . one thing that was missing when Mrs. Erickson and Dr. Erickson drove to Arizona, if in fact they did, was that they didn't have cruise control in those days. No cruise control. Cruise control is such a nice way to drive. You just turn on the cruise control and sit back and steer . . . . the car . . .

JOHN: . . . just notice all the sounds that go by . . .

JULIE: . . . the scenery changes . . .

JOHN: . . . children playing . . .

JULIE: . . . in fact your feet can just relax, because it's just your hand . . . on the steering wheel . . . driving the car, but are you really the one driving and at what rate are you driving? And how many signs would you need to go past until you signal your intentions of . . . *changing* lanes . . .

JOHN: . . . it's always good to signal your intentions . . .

JULIE: . . . before . . .

JOHN: . . . **you change** . . .

JULIE: . . . lanes of traffic. Now if Mrs. Erickson and Dr. Erickson had cruise control . . . you know you don't put on cruise control when you're in a busy city or busy town. You wait until you get out on the high . . . way, and then you turn on the cruise control . . . when you can drive whatever speed you want. Probably the cars back then weren't quite as safe as they would be now, so you can drive quite safely at whatever speed you choose, because they're reinforced now, they're well built, they're solid . . . cars . . .

JOHN: . . . In Phoenix, their destination, the climate was very different, the scenery was different . . .

JULIE: . . . the signs were different . . .

JOHN: . . . and it takes just a little while to adjust . . .

JULIE: . . . people there still *signal the same way* . . . up . . . down . . . left . . right . . . the signals were still the same, the signs were different . . .

JOHN: . . . so there they were . . .

JULIE: . . . as they arrived, they noticed something that they had never seen before . . . It was a particular sign that they saw as they drove into Phoenix . . . something that led them to believe that they were on the right road, going in the right direction . . . as they signaled their intentions about moving . . . to Phoenix . . .

JOHN: . . . until finally, they reached their destination. Time flew by—it can do that when you're in . . . . that's right . . . a different state . . . and they finally arrived at 17 Hayward Avenue,[16] we're told . . and there Betty and Milton stood, motionless, just looking at their new home. If you've ever been in Phoenix, you know many of the homes are adobe looking, with red tile roofs. You could almost say they look the same from the outside . . . even though there are a lot of different things happening inside.

Anyway, there they are looking at this house, and beside it was this reconverted garage. Betty looked at Milton (we're not sure if this is really true) but as the story goes, she looked at Milton and she said, "You know, Milton, that house looks fine, but the garage— we've got to do something about that." Milton said, "What do you mean?" She said, "Look at that garage. There's so much junk that's in the garage. Look at all that junk that's in the garage." Milton looked around, peered through the windows and said, "Yeah, you're right." And she said, "Milton, if we're going to make this our home, the first thing you need to do is you need to get all the junk outside the garage, just get rid of it, get all the junk out." Milton said, "You're right. The thing is . . . it's everybody else's junk, it's not even ours." And they proceeded to *go ahead and get rid of all the junk.*

Now, we really don't know how far the house was from the garage . . . we've heard different stories about this . . . Some people say

What Do Driving And Garages Have To Do With Intention And Trance? 27

that the house is maybe *thirty* feet from the garage, but you never know about these reports. Some said they were already connected ... what's five feet, one way or the other ... it could have easily been *twenty-five* feet to the garage ... another five feet, who knows, that would make it, that's right, about *twenty* feet from the garage ... and as you proceed about another five feet, you get to ...

JULIE: ... deeper and deeper ...

JOHN: ... *fifteen* ...

JULIE: ... just let your own conscious mind rest ... as you go as deeply as you like ...

JOHN: ... you notice something's happening ...

JULIE: ... relax ...

JOHN: ... and you see the threshold of the door ...

JULIE: ... secure ...

JOHN: ... leading *inside* the garage ...

JULIE: ... relax, think ...

JOHN: ... and that garage is the place ...

JULIE: ... enjoy ...

JOHN: ... where Milton had done his life's work...

JULIE: ... purpose ...

JOHN: ... most of his seminars of his later years were done *inside* the garage ... much of the therapy ...

JULIE: ... inside ...

JOHN: ... that occurred, occurred inside ...

JULIE: ... the storehouse ...

JOHN:	. . . the garage . . .
JULIE:	. . . of all things . . .
JOHN:	. . . being a good student walking toward the garage . . .
JULIE:	. . . easily . . .
JOHN:	. . . one would have to be getting curious . . .
JULIE:	. . . very curious . . .
JOHN:	. . . about what it was like to step inside . . .
JULIE:	. . . wondering . . .
JOHN:	. . . *ten* feet . . .
JULIE:	. . . what it would look like inside . . .
JOHN:	. . . all the way in . . .
JULIE:	. . . how would it feel . . .
JOHN:	. . . *five* feet . . .
JULIE:	. . . what would I find inside the garage? . . .
JOHN:	. . . garage . . . and be*fore* you know it, you pass *three* and you *too* are *one* . . .
JULIE:	. . . foot . . .
JOHN:	. . . from being **inside** the garage . . . *Now,* stepping *inside,* at first it seems as though it's dark because it takes a while for your eyes to **make the adjustment** . . .
JULIE:	. . . adjust . . . just go right ahead and adjust . . .
JOHN:	. . . to see clearly in front . . .

JULIE: . . . very clearly . . .

JOHN: . . . and you notice . . .

JULIE: . . . clearer perhaps than you've ever seen . . .

JOHN: . . . what's really inside . . .

JULIE: . . . before . . .

JOHN: . . . and Milton would be there one time or another . . .

JULIE: . . . observing . . .

JOHN: . . . telling . . .

JULIE: . . . magnifying . . .

JOHN: . . . you know it is okay . . .

JULIE: . . . to amplify . . .

JOHN: . . . to trust . . .

JULIE: . . . your powers . . .

JOHN: . . . your unconscious . . .

JULIE: . . . of observation . . .

JOHN: . . . now . . .

JULIE: . . . so that you do . . .

(Someone's book slides off their lap and onto the floor.)

JOHN: . . . remove all the old constructs . . .

JULIE: . . . just fall away, let them all go . . .

JOHN: . . . just letting it go . . .

JULIE: . . . toss them aside, throw the junk out, it wasn't yours to begin with . . .

JOHN: . . . and there it was inside, all these books . . .

JULIE: . . . loads of books . . .

JOHN: . . . and all kinds of pictures . . .

JULIE: . . . memorabilia . . .

JOHN: . . . so many memories inside . . .

JULIE: . . . trinkets . . .

JOHN: . . . things that were gifts from other people . . .

JULIE: . . . wood carvings . . .

JOHN: . . . little mementoes that different people had left there . . .

JULIE: . . . a purple telephone . . .

JOHN: . . . different people . . .

JULIE: . . . a purple octopus . . .

JOHN: . . . all sorts of things inside the garage . . .

JULIE: . . . many things, but all things that meant something, mean even more inside . . .

JOHN: . . . because he always wanted you to know . . . to take the time you need inside, so that you really can *trust your unconscious* . . . mind . . . knows all that you need to know . . .

JULIE: . . . so that you can be just as excited as a little child to *trust your unconscious mind* and enjoy your unconscious processes . . .

JOHN: . . . and he'd often say that you are all here for a reason . . .

What Do Driving And Garages Have To Do With Intention And Trance? 31

JULIE: . . . and you are all here for a reason . . . we don't know perhaps the full scope of the reason why you are here . . . you, too, may not know that . . . consciously . . . yet . . .

JOHN: . . . and whether it was stated explicitly . . .

JULIE: . . . and your unconscious brought you . . .

JOHN: . . . or it was stated implicitly . . .

JULIE: . . . and your conscious brought you here today to hear what we're saying about hypnosis . . .

JOHN: . . . everyone's present . . .

JULIE: . . . trance . . .

JOHN: . . . inside the garage . . .

JULIE: . . . was there for a reason . . .

JOHN: . . . to become ultimately as accomplished as Milton, in your own particular way, in your own particular style, with your own particular personality, with your own particular gifts that you have to offer . . .

JULIE: . . . because not only was Erickson a great hypnotherapist, he was also a great trance subject himself . . .

JOHN: . . . one of the things that a good trance subject knows . . .

JULIE: . . . all good trance subjects have higher intelligence . . .

JOHN: . . . is how it's possible . . .

JULIE: . . . they all know certain things . . .

JOHN: . . . to follow certain suggestions that are appropriate . . .

JULIE: . . . easily and comfortably . . .

JOHN: . . . for your unconscious . . .

JULIE: . . . and they do better and better . . .

JOHN: . . . because one of Milton's favorite suggestions was in a little bit, not yet, but in a little bit, I'd like you to go ahead and open your eyes and feel as though you have awakened, taking all the time that you need, that's right . . .

JULIE: . . . but when you open your eyes, you can notice that you can let your body sleep, so that your eyes can awaken, but your body is still resting . . .

JOHN: . . . in a driving trance . . .

JULIE: . . . a driving trance . . .

JOHN: . . . where your eyes are open . . .

JULIE: . . . always keep your eyes open . . .

JOHN: . . . and you can see where you are going . . .

JULIE: . . . when you're on the high . . . way . . .

JOHN: . . . you know how to signal your intentions . . .

JULIE: . . . see the signs, signal your intentions . . . drive the speed you want to go at . . . It's safe. So in a moment you can open your eyes, but let your body stay relaxed so you as a mind you can be here, and your body can be elsewhere, just resting . . . while we continue with the training.

Begin to reorient.

The Four Keys To Doing Ericksonian Work And Being Certifiable!

Now we know that some of you are very serious about becoming exquisite Ericksonian Hypnotherapists. So these are the four keys for being certifiable and doing Ericksonian work! (Yes, we're serious about being tongue in cheek.)

Number one, we know some of you already follow suggestions very well

. . . that's right. As Cindy has already said, the first key is to wear lots of purple. If you need to update your wardrobe, fashion consultants are standing by!

The second requirement to be certifiable and to do Ericksonian work is to *speak* in a low, gravelly, *hypnotic* voice.

The third key is that you have to say, *"That's right."*

"That's Right" Exercise

We've got an exercise we want you to do. Some of your bodies are still asleep . . . that's totally okay . . . we know who you are . . . because you know how it's possible to walk in your sleep . . . of course, the name of this exercise is . . . (group answers) "That's right!" . . . here's what we'll do. There will be three people . . . an A, a B, and a C.

This is one of these exercises which will challenge you significantly! Particularly if you're B. We'll start with B. B, your job is to do the following, (now just fasten your seat belts on this one) *just sit there* and B (be), okay? Now A is going to look at B, and notice that B is just sitting there. Before A does anything else, A is going to make a representation in his or her mind which will be the foundation of this training. A is going to hold three beliefs about B in his/her mind to direct and align their intention. The first belief about B is: *"You are a great hypnotic subject."* So you're going to make a picture in your mind of B being a great hypnotic subject. You're then going to include the belief (as you're saying this to B in your mind), *"You are totally resourceful"* and the third belief that you'll be holding is: *"You can change easily and timely."*

Take a few moments to create a picture in your mind of that person with all of the qualities which would be present in someone who personifies these beliefs:

YOU'RE A GREAT HYPNOTIC SUBJECT
YOU ARE TOTALLY RESOURCEFUL
YOU CAN CHANGE EASILY AND TIMELY

Make arrangements for your unconscious mind to hold these beliefs in the back of your mind during the entire time you do this exercise.

Then whenever A observes B doing anything at all which they would consider to be trance, you know what A is going to say, don't you? "That's right . . . that's right . . . that's right." That's all A is going to do. A will look at B meaningfully, and say "That's right" whenever they see B do any behavior which looks like trance. A continues to observe what occurs.

C has the most interesting job of all. C's job is to go into an "uptime," or outside trance, which we're going to teach you. (See APPENDIX) A fast way to access this state is to go into peripheral vision. C's job is, appropriately enough, to "see." So when you're C, you see . . . the relationship between A and B. When C sees A and B form a hypnotic relationship, then C will begin to nod hypnotically. Now, do you know how to nod hypnotically? This is nodding hypnotically (nods very slowly and cataleptically). You continue to do that as long as you observe that the relationship between A and B is hypnotic.

This is a thirty-minute exercise with ten minutes per round, so everyone will have the opportunity to be in each role. We'll give you the signal at the end of ten minutes to *change* roles. Notice you can stay in this state because Pennsylvania is too big to leave at this point. Quietly remaining in the state, ready, go!

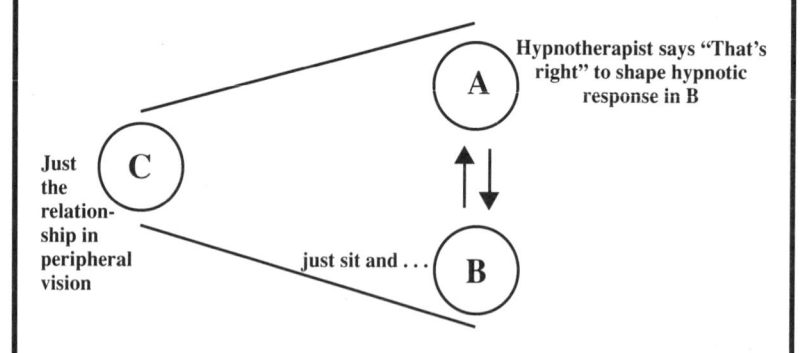

Figure 2.2 The "That's Right" exercise. This exercise is designed to create trance in each position. However, the trance state for each position is different. The function of the respective roles (A, B, or C) determines the difference in the trance.

Do the exercise

What Do Driving And Garages Have To Do With Intention And Trance?

Discussion

What you just learned in this exercise was something that took Dr. Erickson many years to understand, and this understanding changed the field of hypnotherapy. Later in his career, he said, "My learning over the years was that I tried to direct the patient too much. It took me a long time to *let things develop* and make use of things as they developed."[17]

So how many of you noticed that was . . . a . . . deep experience? . . . . . . Only the people who can still raise their hands! . . . . . . Cataleptically, that's right. First of all, any observations—any questions?

PAUL: Since my client (because of the order in which we did this) already held the belief that she was a great hypnotic subject, I found that if I simply matched and mirrored her, I'd be a great hypnotherapist!

Very good observation; because one of our covert goals was to install the idea that if you really believe your clients are great hypnotic subjects, and you follow them, you will be, by presupposition, a great hypnotherapist yourself. The reason that's true is because hypnosis is a cybernetic relationship.

JACQUELINE: By doing this content-free, I had the opportunity to notice I was doing a lot of matching and mirroring on a physiological level which I hadn't been aware of before.

Not consciously aware of before. This exercise is useful because we've isolated the external trance behaviors of your client so you will be paying attention to those consciously. You can make any associations necessary with the new information and then let go of it consciously and allow it to become unconscious again. A significant portion of our growth as hypnotherapists comes from exercises or experiences like this where you pull out something which is typically unconscious and make it conscious. You can then evaluate it, make any necessary adjustments, and then return it to the unconscious mind. When you return it to the unconscious, it returns there with the addition of your new experience and learnings.

PATRICE: I noticed when I was A, I was not in trance as deeply as when I was B and C.

Excellent observation . . . so you noticed all three positions involved trance, which means you had about thirty minutes to experience different levels of trance. Every position you were in, whether you were A, B or C, was trance. There were different qualities to each of the trances, because you were paying attention to different information depending on your role. So it's probably appropriate that you were not as deeply in trance when you were A because you were the hypnotherapist then. The hypnotherapist's trance is an uptime trance in contrast to the client's which is a downtime trance.

What you've commented on so far is in alignment philosophically with what we were hoping you would get and that is all people have their own way of doing trance. Each person goes into and experiences trance differently. One of the reasons why Erickson was so successful, relative to some of his contemporaries, was simply because he took anything he considered to be an unconscious response as an indication of trance development. He was like a kid in a candy shop. Anything he saw which he thought presupposed trance was useful to him. "Oh, they're blinking! That's great! Their breathing shifted, that's great! Their eyes have closed!" . . . and so on.

Think about the effect that this would have on you, to be part of a hypnotic system and *every time you see certain nonverbals you're feeling more and more confident of what's happening*. Your feelings of confidence are going to be transmitted to the person that you're working with in the hypnosis session. The realization that people can go into trance with their eyes open, their eyes closed, while they're standing on their feet, or while they're sitting down is very reassuring for the hypnotherapist. The client can go into trance doing all sorts of behaviors and your job is simply to observe when they are displaying trance behaviors. Catch them being in trance and utilize that.

Erickson also said he noticed he would vary the trance behaviors to which he paid attention. He would follow one indicator as far as possible then he would switch. One of the things most people who begin doing hypnosis aren't aware of is that very rarely does a person go into a deep trance and stay at that level without shifting their consciousness to other levels. If their clients open their eyes or shift in their chair, the therapist might become discouraged and think, "Oh, this person is not in trance anymore." While in trance, people cycle through different levels of experience. Sometimes they will be in a light trance, sometimes in a deep trance, and sometimes they will be somewhere in between both extremes. Erickson often said that people can be in a light trance and a deep trance simultaneously.[18] They can be deeply engaged in what is being said and at the same time be aware of other things going on in the room and in their external environment. The whole issue of depth is a metaphor, and there are many places where metaphors are limited. In this case, it's better to have other ways to gauge trance than by depth alone.

Erickson advocated assisting others to experience a "sufficient" trance. The question is: "What is a sufficient trance?" Well, it's whatever state the subject needs to be in to get the job done. When you see people floating or cycling in and out of trance, that's fine. We do that naturally as we sleep. We don't stay in Stage Four sleep, which looks similar to being comatose, the whole time we're sleeping. While you're dreaming, you're actually very active and you would be extremely active physiologically if you didn't have the voluntary muscle inhibition reflex. When you come out of a dream in the middle of the night, you're very close to waking up. This would also be the time when people would have to go to the bathroom, or they would shift around before they cycle back down again. Our neurology is based upon naturally occurring cycles, and trance also appears to occur in natural cycles.

As we mentioned earlier, we all have ultradian rhythms which occur every 90-120 minutes.[19] One of the implications of these rhythms is that during waking hours your mind will spontaneously take a break within this time frame. Switching to something else temporarily allows your mind to integrate whatever is going on. At least every 120 minutes, and for some people it happens as early as 90 minutes into the cycle, the unconscious will provide a neurological break. If you just catch your client when they're in one of those trances and utilize it, you'll assist them in going into trance very easily.

PAUL: Sometimes I go a little too far out, and I'm not sure I know what the task is.

Ah ha, a trance junkie! So you're going inside instead of staying in an uptime or outside trance. It would be valuable for you to <u>consciously</u> practice the peripheral vision technique so you develop the kinesthetics and a recognition of those kinesthetics which accompany an external focus. An uptime trance, where your focus is on something external (the client, sounds, the trainer's voice, etc.), is the best trance state for being in the hypnotherapist's role. A downtime trance, where your focus is inward, is useful when you are the client, when you're meditating, or perhaps when you are listening to a therapeutic changework tape. Trance is generally useful in any context. What's important is practicing both variations, so your neurology is flexible enough to shift your attention from inside to outside, or vice versa, at a moment's notice, depending on what's required in the specific context.

Whether the trances you utilize are uptime or downtime states, it is important to find balance inside yourself between your conscious and your unconscious mind. That's a metaphor for life. How well you live your life may be a delicate balance between your conscious and unconscious processing.

Creating Positive Internal Representations

In wrapping up the exercise, we'd like to take a moment and discuss in more detail the notion of holding positive internal representations of ourselves and others.

Most of you who have been at this for a while know that, in most cases, the unconscious mind does not easily process negation. The word "not" or any of its derivatives only exists in the world of language. Therefore, you can't not think about what it is you don't want to think about without thinking about it first . . . . . . Think about that . . . or not . . . ! This means your unconscious functions far more smoothly when you are concentrating on what you want as opposed to what you don't want. This principle is closely related to a "law" in the field of Hypnosis called the "Law of Reverse Effect," which states that the more you *try* not to think about something, the more you will think about it.[20] Further, it's useful to consider whether the internal representations, or the intention, which you have for your clients is empowering to them. Our complex equivalence for internal representation is our intention. Clearly, from our research, virtually every spiritual system teaches its aspirants to see God or the goodness in everyone, and our intention is to do that. To the extent that we do, we assist others in doing that for themselves.

It has been very personally meaningful for me to hold the internal representation of exactly how I want the person to be when I'm interacting with them. In a particular training a few years ago, we did an experiment to test this. We asked the therapists to see their clients fully experiencing their outcome as the client was asked to present the problem. We then asked the client to discuss the problem, inviting them to "try" to hold onto it as the therapist just listened and held a totally positive, resourceful image in their mind. The most common experience was as the client talked about the problem, they began to run out of steam and were left a bit bemused that what they were discussing even seemed like a problem in the first place!

You see, people around us can only function as well as our filters allow. If we hold an unresourceful representation of another, chances are we'll filter out that which is inconsistent with our internal representation. Since relationships are cybernetic, those same representations are going to govern our behavior toward others as well as influence how we interpret feedback. When you add in the concept of "perception is projection," then positive internal representations are affecting us at another level simultaneously. If we're holding a less-than-magnificent image of others, we might ask, "Whose neurology is it wired to and therefore whose is it effecting?"

This may be what it all boils down to. The techniques give <u>you</u> something to do, so when the client comes to see you, <u>they</u> know that you're doing something! Techniques appeal to their conscious mind, giving it something to think about. They also structure the unconscious mind, not only of the client, but also, we believe, of the therapist, which allows the healing to take place. As practitioners of NLP and Hypnosis, after you practice the techniques well enough, they become part of the repertoire of your unconscious mind. So when you're holding the belief that you're working with a great hypnotic subject, and you know how to do the techniques, you can really assist the client in achieving their outcomes. Your internal representation and the techniques work together synergistically.

For every exercise, before you begin to work with someone, the first thing we want you to do is to make a representation in your mind of your client with the three beliefs we described or seeing them fully experiencing their outcome. That will allow you to do the things which we were discussing and it will also mobilize your unconscious mind to do what you can to support those representations. If you see someone as basically "insensitive" (or any other negative representation), then what's going to happen is your unconscious mind will send messages to your body to behave in a way which supports that particular association and guess what? . . . . . . You'll get to be right! The question is: "Would you rather be right or would you rather have a relationship that works?" If you'd rather have a relationship which works and works well, hold onto the positive intention, then once again you'll be right.

This is the end of this section, and we really don't need to make a direct suggestion that it's time to turn the page yet, because we haven't reminded you of all the other times in your life where you were *learning something meaningful* and you may have enjoyed pausing to *collect your thoughts, shift* in your chair, or acquire something delicious to eat or drink. Who knows what you want to do right now or how soon you'll actualize that behavior, perhaps you won't know the answer until you DO turn the page NOW!! . . . . . . Any other suggestions?

Chapter 3
Structuring Trance Inductions, Naturally

Editor's Notes: If Chapter One and Two are the appetizers, then Chapter Three marks the beginning of several main courses. Chapters Three through Six represent the core ingredients of the trainers' modeling project. Chapter Seven, which includes the Hypnotic Interview, is a synthesis of these chapters.

The purpose of this chapter is to go beyond the setup, as the participants have by now been going in and out of trance for several hours. Revivification and Pacing Current Experience, two of Erickson's most frequently used inductions, are the topics of conversation. The trainers also share one of the easiest ways <u>ever</u> to elicit trance (page 50-51); it is extremely conversational and nearly foolproof.

Readers are referred to the demonstrations, virtually all of which are verbatim transcripts from the actual recording. They offer a brilliant exposition of how easily Revivification and Pacing Current Experience can be blended and anchored together, as well as providing excellent examples of hypnotic language patterns. This chapter also ends with a brief question-and-answer segment.

The italicized references denote when the trainers use hypnotic voice analogs. The reader may be interested in reading only these references at some point to determine what message they convey.

What would a hypnosis training be without trance inductions? *Naturally, we hope these inductions will be a trans-parent model, guiding you to a deeper understanding of unconscious communication.* In the next two chapters, we're going to survey the structures, popularized by Erickson, for doing hypnotic inductions. In this chapter, we will start with **Revivification** and **Pacing Current Experience.** In the following chapter, we will cover **Conscious-Unconscious Dissociation.** In a later section, we will integrate these inductions into a comprehensive approach. In clinical practice, there is often no real delineation between these techniques because they are blended and layered together. The value of interweaving these inductions is not only to deepen trance, but to deepen unconscious rapport.

It's beneficial to remember that these inductions are to assist you in structuring the context so your client can be free to *pay attention to what is immediately important* in making their desired change. Whether or not you *memorize these structures* is not nearly as important as your ability to *grasp the spirit of cooperation* inherent in them.

Revivification

Erickson often appeared to simply carry on casual conversations with his clients. He would talk to them about a prior experience and begin to develop it by either asking questions or simply hallucinating general, universal elements for the experience. The greater the amount of detail he requested, the more deeply associated to the experience the client would become. Some clients would *virtually relive* the memory in the present moment. This simple yet elegant process for creating trance is referred to as Revivification.

Revivification is very useful because you can utilize it before you begin the "changework" or the "trance induction." It's so innocuous. You could just ask the person: "Do you have any hobbies or what do you do in your spare time?" This is an example for those with a background in NLP, where you can use and ought to use the Meta Model[1] to induce trance. Generally the Milton Model is considered to be the model that induces trance. The Milton Model facilitates trance when you don't know about the client's internal experience. By being meaningfully ambiguous in language, it prompts the recipient to go inside and access their own personal history, to make sense of what has been said to them.

On the other hand, if you ask them questions and they tell you about their internal experience, the more detailed questions you ask, the more likely you'll be installing that state as you're asking the questions. They'll have to access the particular file for that memory, open it, and stay in it to answer the questions. This process will necessarily alter their time-space orientation. In working with clients, you want to be clear about what you are installing. If you're going to chunk down into the details about certain experiences, it will generally be far more expeditious to do this with positive experiences. Once you have revivified a positive experience, you can anchor[2] the feelings associated with it and use these as resources later in the therapy session. (There's no real reason to revivify negative experiences, because most clients have little difficulty accessing the problem, and all you really need to know is the structure of the problem. In fact, revivifying a negative experience could potentially anchor them into an unresourceful state and compound the negative feelings or trauma.)

One of the things Erickson did (and this can be thought of as a series of "mini" trances) was to ask a person about several different experiences in one conversation. He may have asked about a hobby, a recent vacation, or their family life. As he talked to them, he assisted them in revivifying those memories, so they would experience the accompanying emotions in the therapy session. Later he would use a phrase or word which would reactivate the association to those feelings. To an outside observer, all he was doing was carrying on a pleasant conversation. However, this "casual" conversation accomplished a number of important objectives: it facilitated rapport (most people like to talk about hobbies, pleasant memories, etc.); it provided the therapist with visual and auditory feedback regarding the client's responsiveness; it began to train the client in trance; and it uncovered potential resources for later use.

General Steps To Revivification

The first step while establishing rapport (matching and mirroring physiology and auditory qualities) is to ask general questions which direct the client toward hobbies, vacations, or pleasant occurrences on the job or with their family. At this point, it will appear that you're getting a brief history and an overall sense of how your client spends time.

Second, once you've found an area which may have resourceful states associated with it, start asking Meta Model questions. These are questions designed to gather specific, detailed information. You'll begin by asking questions which are external, contextual questions such as: when, where, with whom or what was happening? These questions will orient the person to the context. You ought to be calibrating to their physiology to notice how intense the state is and how fully they are accessing it. Once you begin to notice that they are oriented to the context, change your tense from past to present tense. Use linkage words like "as," "and," "while," etc., to create smooth and fluid transitions. For example, "When you think about that great training you attended (dissociated past tense), what is (requesting associated present tense) the most intense part?........(Wait for response.)........ And as that is happening ..... what are you feeling now?"

Continue chunking down, but begin directing the client's attention inward to his or her sensations, feelings, and thoughts at the time. This does several things: it intensifies the kinesthetics because bringing attention inward will generally initiate trance development; and the client will be more likely to verbalize "loaded words" complete with the nonverbal analogs which are naturalistic anchors for that experience.

In NLP terms, this process is the elicitation of their reality strategy. The primary question used to elicit reality strategies is: "How do you know?" For example, a client might begin to tell you about a feeling of expansiveness. You would ask: "How do you know you're feeling expansive? Where do you feel it?" The client replies, "I feel it all through my chest." By asking these questions, you're "chunking down" and getting more details about how they know an experience is real for them.

As you ask them questions like, "Where were you when it happened?" use your conversational voice. For example they might say, "I was at school." You might respond, "Oh, you were at school. When was this in school?" "I was a senior in high school." "You were at school and you were a senior in high school." Then as you continue, progressively slow down your voice, lower your pitch, and begin modeling trance. "What was actually happening that makes it such a deep experience?" "The teacher just kept droning on and on." "The teacher just kept droning on and on." "The more that they kept talking, the more my mind just went away." "So the more they talked, the more your mind just went away. How do you know you're in a trance?" "I feel my body sinking into the chair." "Your body just sinks into the chair. What else?" "My mind just sort of goes away." "Your mind gooooes a . . . . way."

Once you have the reality strategy, elicit a loaded word or phrase that captures the state, repeat it back in trance analogs (physiology and tonality which matches trance) and remember it for future use. For example, in the Monde tapes[3,4] Erickson asks Monde to find a happy experience. She finds a time when she was two years old and splashing in the water. He refers to that as "two year old Monde . . . splashing in the water."[5] That's his anchor for that state. Later in the therapy, at just the right moment, he uses this particular phrase as an auditory anchor for the resourceful emotions he wants her to experience.

The final step is to provide the suggestion: "Open your eyes only as quickly as your unconscious mind is prepared to deepen (anchor word or key phrase) the next time you access it." If their eyes haven't closed as you were eliciting the reality strategy, just tell them how much more they can enjoy the experience after their eyes are closed (while you model eye closure by doing a prolonged blink yourself). Only they'll know how much more enjoyment they will have once they close their eyes.

Demonstration of Revivification

JOHN: Who would be willing to sit up here and have a positive deep trance experience?

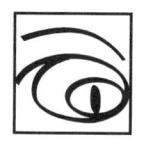

Okay, Cindy, come on up. (To audience.) You may notice that most of the time we like to do demos standing. I'm also doing that today because I want all of you to realize that if your client is sitting and you're standing, you can still be in rapport with them. There are many other things you can match and mirror to establish rapport.

Okay, Cindy, how are you doing up here, you're doing okay? I don't know what it's like for you to be sitting up here. I don't know if there have been times in your life, maybe a specific time, when you had a positive deep trance experience. You have? I was wondering, where were you?

CINDY: Probably the time I remember most was when I was here in the spring.

JOHN: (Repeats back) You were here in this room. In the spring? And how were you seated?

CINDY: In one of those chairs, with my legs relaxed.

JOHN: Legs relaxed. Mmm. Mmmm. What was actually happening at the time causing you to have a deep trance?

CINDY: Ted and I were doing the "That's Right" exercise.

JOHN: The "That's Right" exercise. So you were just hearing someone say "That's right."

CINDY: Real soothing.

JOHN: And when do you begin to notice you're going (present tense) into trance the whole way? What are you feeling?

CINDY: Warm. Very Warm.

JOHN: Warm. Very warm. Feeling the warmth where?

CINDY: Everywhere...

JOHN: That's right. **Warm** ...... everywhere .... As you're feeling warm everywhere...noticing how you experience the sensations in your body.... I don't know just how much better you can feel inside .. warmth ... that's right .... as deeply as you do ... now ... since you volunteered to do this as well as you have, I'd like to just suggest ... that's right ... that not only will your eyes open, you will have them open only as quickly as your unconscious mind can deepen that experience the next time you access it and that will allow you to experience another time that you haven't thought of just yet ... similar in intensity .... that can add to the intensity of your current trance .... Only allow your eyes to open as quickly as you can deepen that experience ... That's right! .... Warm (the anchor) ... the next time you access it ...... Now ..!

(Cindy begins to open her eyes, but the rest of her body remains quite still and fixed. She turns her head slightly to look at the trainer.)

Welcome back. How you doing? Pretty simple, huh? Was it a nice experience?

CINDY: Am I done?

JOHN: Are you? (To the audience.) Because she's still coming out of trance, she needs to understand literally what the next set of instructions is. Right now she's sitting here and she doesn't know what to do. This is a great time to make a suggestion, which can be incorporated into whatever the experience was that she just had. So as long as I talk like this (soft, trance voice), she'll remain in trance. If I start to talk like this (conversational voice), now she'll know I'm done. I wasn't talking like this was I? (conversational voice) I was talking more quietly in a trance voice (soft, trance voice.) That's right. Do you see the skin color change as soon as I start to change my voice? Right up in here. (Trainer looks at Cindy and speaks in a conversational voice) Okay? ...

CINDY: Yep. (Moves her body, shifts and then begins to get out of the chair.)

JOHN: Great job! .... Give her a hand.

Discussion

One of the things which I was tempted to do with Cindy and didn't was arm catalepsy. Both of her arms were quite fixed and rigidly resting on the arms of the chair. Either of her arms could have been easily lifted and would have remained suspended cataleptically. Catalepsy is balanced tonicity in the muscles between agonist and antagonist muscles. In Cindy's case it was a "waxy flexibility," or a certain rigidity, in the muscles of her arms. We didn't utilize it yet because we're not teaching that right now.

A second point related to Cindy's demo is what you might say when you observe your client is still partially in trance at the end of the exercise: **"You're a great hypnotic subject."** If a client is still partially in trance and you have some time to allow them to orient, this is a great opportunity to make further suggestions which support the efficacy of the trance or you can utilize this as an opportunity to reinduce trance, a technique called fractionation. In the presence of rapport, going in and out of a series of trances tends to deepen the succeeding trance. This is a great way to work with a naive client (a technical term denoting one who has not formally experienced trance). It gently trains their neurology.

There is also another anchor operating here, other than the obvious one which you used to revivify the experience, and that is your voice tonality. You want people to *understand* when you're talking to their conscious mind and when you're talking to their (lowers voice pitch into hypnotic voice and looks directly at Dot) *unconscious* mind. So you *begin* to do what Erickson called the interspersal technique[6] where you *drop* in certain embedded commands . . . . (Dot's eyes briefly flutter and begin to close.)
. . . *Good* . . . . *That's good, Dot* . . . .*Very good.* **You're a great hypnotic subject.**

(Returning to discussion with the rest of the class about Cindy's demo.)

Did you also notice how brief it can be? Cindy accessed the trance and we could see it happening as her breathing shifted, her head came down, and she went inside. Did you notice that only a few questions were necessary? In fact, the fewer questions you ask, the better, because it will more closely resemble normal conversation. You can either do it very briefly or if you'd like to experiment, you can ask for more details. The easiest way to know is to just calibrate to your client and see how deeply they go into trance. They only need to be in the state long enough for you to set an anchor and for them to come back outside. It might take as little as one minute to do this, even seconds. I stretched it out for demonstration purposes, and also, because it was a

48 TRAINING TRANCES

trance state which I was eliciting. When you're eliciting trance, you generally want to provide the subject with enough time to access a comfortably light to medium trance. We may choose to elicit trance with a more formal induction, but it's more fun to start combining techniques, as we shall see.

Now here's an important key to increasing your effectiveness in any induction that you do. When you speak to your client, **look** at them ***meaningfully and expectantly.*** And what are we expecting? We are expecting they are going to access the desired state. After all, they're a great hypnotic subject. This process may also be used to revivify states other than trance. Revivification may be used for any state which would be useful in the therapeutic context, such as: curiosity, confidence, security, anticipation, etc. Since this is a training in trance, we're using Revivification to recreate trance here.

Everybody got it? Lets take ten minutes each, twenty minutes total. When you're finished with this part of the exercise, we'll add another layer to it. This is a progressive exercise. You'll be utilizing the anchor you set in this exercise in the next exercise also.

Revivification Exercise

1. Match and mirror physiology while asking general questions about a positive deep trance experience.

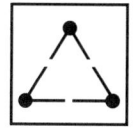

   Look at your client meaningfully and expectantly.

2. Use Meta Model questions to elicit specifics about an experience:
   a. when, where, with whom.
   b. use conjunctions to create smooth transitions.
   c. change tense from past to present.
   d. direct focus from external to internal.

3. Begin repeating verbal and nonverbal responses and begin to lead and model trance physiology as you continue the dialogue. If necessary ask, "How do you know you're in a trance?"

4. Identify a key word or phrase that captures the state:
   a. include trance analogs.
   b. remember the phrase!

5. Give posthypnotic suggestion:
   "Open your eyes only as quickly as your unconscious mind is prepared to deepen (<u>anchor</u> <u>word</u> or <u>key</u> <u>phrase</u>), the next time you access it."

Do the exercise

Welcome back. Now here's something to consider. Can you begin to get a sense of using this as a "starter" trance induction where you have maybe three to four other experiences you've revivified and anchored? Yet as far as your client's concerned, you haven't even started "Hypnosis." You didn't ask them to find a point on the wall, fixate their attention, or any of those "hypnotic things."

At this point, you have these states anchored so they're readily available as resources for your client to *make changes*. Then when you actually do the "real" trance induction, it will go very smoothly because you'll have everything set up in advance. We'll continue using this approach of sequencing and anchoring when we teach you the metaphor intervention we modeled from Erickson's work. (Briefly, a series of metaphors are done first without "formally" establishing trance. After the metaphors are anchored, then you do the "formal" trance induction. You then fire the anchors sequentially from all the metaphors during the formal induction . . . but don't consider this fully because we're not there yet!)

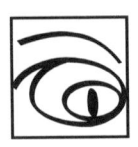

Demonstration of Reality Strategy To Suspend Belief And Induce Trance

(Trainer looks at Dot still seated in the audience.)

Trainer: Dot, do you think you're in a trance right now?

DOT: I think so . . . .

Trainer: How do you know that? Your body just went . . . What specifically lets you know that you are . . . or aren't you sure *you're really in a deep trance?* Are you in a ***deep*** *trance,* now?

DOT: (Shakes her head) No . . . . I don't think so.

Trainer: You don't . . . think . . . . so . . . . how would you know that *you are in a deep trance* even though you don't think so?

DOT: (Eyes fixed straight ahead, body motionless) My body . . . . . .

Trainer: Your body. What about your body? . . . . Even though you don't think so . . . . What about your body?

DOT: I wouldn't feel my body . . . . (voice is noticeably softer, articulation is slow and monotone).

Trainer: That's right. You don't feel your body . . . (matches her voice) . . . That's right. All the way . . . . (model eye closure) . . . . Very good, Dot . . . . And you can float as a mind while your body is down there.
 And notice what you can *learn from the point of view of being a mind and seeing all that's happening while your body's down there, learning what you've learned about this particular hypnotic communication. So that you, too, your conscious and unconscious will*

*have the same ability to replicate this and to do this with someone else and only as quickly as you begin to come back outside and **open your eyes** . . . . Take all the time you need, Dot, to do it comfortably and easily . . . . All the way out, right.*

(To audience) Do you understand the value of getting the person's reality strategy? Because either response they offer is perfect. If you ask, "Do you think you're in a trance?" and the person says, "I don't think so," that's great. If they say "I don't think so," what part of their brain, in terms of hemispheres, is not working the way it normally does? There is some question in their mind, isn't there? So their consciousness is already beginning to shift over to the subdominant hemisphere. All you do then is play it back and say, "Oh, you don't think so." Now the person is questioning, "Am I . . . in a trance?" Once they experience that moment of uncertainty or confusion, that's the doorway to trance. Then all I have to do is give a couple of other suggestions and in Dot's case, she went "whump," right into trance.

It's certainly helpful to sprinkle embedded commands to support the process as well. (Looking at Dot) Plus **you're a great hypnotic subject.** Have you felt your body just yet? You are a great trance subject . . . . (To audience) Look at her arms and the way she's sitting there. She hasn't moved them. (To Dot) It's okay to move your arms, Dot, whenever you're ready . . . that will help . . . (To audience and Dot) Okay, there's a bit of motion. Notice for the most part she hasn't fully shifted yet. Part of her is still in trance and that's okay. She needs to take the time she wants because she's learning to dissociate, which is a very useful process. (Dot now shifts fully and stretches.)

Pacing Current Experience

This is another structure for inducing trance which Erickson used frequently. In fact, we would be hard pressed to find a time when he didn't use it. What we're calling Pacing Current Experience is the basis for the term he and Ernest Rossi coined as "utilization."[7] The premise is that you always begin with whatever your client presents you. Erickson was quoted as saying that he took every utterance and movement of his clients as a communication to him about their experience.[8]

As you may know, an often-cited precursor to trance is fixation of attention.[9] Traditionally, this was typically done through eye fixation. Eye fixation works well when you're doing a demonstration at a workshop, but in the clinical setting, most clients are already fixated on something else: the problem. Why not use this instead of trying to compete with it by using a stilted protocol to fixate their attention? You just start where they are and go from there.

(Speaking to the audience, some of whom are taking notes and others who are watching and listening.) If you've studied Erickson, you are probably familiar with pacing and leading. As you listen to me—you may want to write this one down—this is the second induction. As you're writing it down, you can begin thinking about how you're actually going to be doing it. (Over the next several sentences, voice tonality gradually changes from conscious teaching voice to hypnotic voice.)

When you look back up here, one of the things you can start to do is begin to consider who you're going to be working with next. As you consider working with that person, what you will be doing is watching what they're doing. As you watch what they're doing, all that you'll do is you'll say to them, "And you're sitting there, listening to what I'm saying . . ." (we're two levels deep now) *" . . . Listening to what I'm saying and beginning to wonder about what we're going to do or maybe you know what we're going to do. You may become aware of certain sensations, maybe the feelings of the backs of your legs against the chair, or maybe just your back against the chair and all those things can help you relax even further. I don't know just how you'll relax, you might relax by just sitting there. You might relax by thinking of some time when you were relaxed, I really don't know."*

That's Pacing Current Experience. Pacing statements are those which are undeniable when the client hears them. Ernest Rossi calls them truisms.[10] Typically when people are taught the technique of Pacing Current Experience, what they're really taught is pacing current **sensory** experience. We'd like to suggest, as a far more elegant way, that you talk about things you know have to be true but aren't necessarily sensory-based.

You might start off with, *"You're sitting there, all of you who have come to this seminar. All of you have come to this seminar with a purpose . . . and fulfilling that purpose is something that can cause you to make changes in your life. After all, that's why you're here. As you listen to what I'm saying right now, you're thinking about what I'm saying. Maybe that's creating other associations in your thinking or maybe you're just continuing to listen to what I'm saying."*

I can say things like, "You came here with a purpose." Well, if they came here, there had to be some purpose. They can't deny that. There's something they want to learn, something they want to know. You can even say, "You don't even realize just yet what your purpose was in coming here." It's artful use of ambiguity with a liberal sprinkling of presuppositions of awareness.

"Perhaps you're not yet **aware** of my using presuppositions of awareness. But you may begin to **notice** them . . . . just **think** about it . . . as you're **paying attention** to what I'm saying, maybe you're not **considering** words like **aware, notice, think, pay attention** or **consider** just yet . . . .

that's right ...... it will become more evident later after you've successfully completed the exercise ..... Not **now** ...... Of course, not **now** ..." (Both trainers simultaneously) ... "Later!"

What is wonderful about presuppositions of awareness is they can create an instant lead from the previous pace. They cause the person who is receiving the communication to follow you with their attention. When you put a "not" in front of the presupposition of awareness, the effect is largely the same: "Perhaps you are not aware of holding this book right now ... because it's far more important to consider what's happening to you right now as you're reading this and maybe you're beginning to realize this truly is a training in trance .... OOOPS ... lost our quotes!

When you pace your partner's or client's experience, you can begin with the circumstances for being there. You can also use behaviors which you know they are doing. If you have a person who's fidgeting, are you going to talk about how they're paying attention to what you're saying? No. You're going to say, "And your mind is moving from one thing to another. You're really not sure what it is that you're thinking about right now and that's really okay. Because you're sitting there, you're leaning back, you're in your chair, you're in this room with me. And if you're here in this room with me, then you've got to hear some of what I'm saying but you can go ahead and let your mind wander all that you like."

What you're doing is providing several paces before you present the lead. A lead refers to the direction in which you want your partner or client to move. In this exercise, we want to move into trance, relaxation, comfort, security, or another similar state.

General Steps To Pacing And Leading

Here's the exercise. Get with the same partner ..... yes, on purpose. In this induction, you're going to use the same nonverbal analogs. In other words, you're going to match and mirror your partner, and you're going to model trance for them while you do the pacing and leading. The easiest way to start this, if you want to do standard pacing and leading, is to utilize the eyeblink reflex. You all know that one, right? So you're sitting there and you're looking at me and your eyes are blinking. Once they're blinking, what do you say?

AUDIENCE: "That's right."

... They <u>are</u> blinking. You isolate one area of behavior and you focus in on that particular area. You then pace and lead that particular behavior. If by following that particular behavior your partner begins to access the state, then you know you want to continue going down that path. If they're not beginning to access the state, then just pick another behavior. There are literally hundreds of different behaviors that they're already doing from which you can choose. In this exercise, your outcome is to assist your partner in accessing a nice, deep trance.

Secondly, once their eyes have closed, you can remind them of that previous positive, deep trance experience with the words you used as anchors in the earlier experience. (We're creating two stages here as we begin to combine both techniques: the first is pacing their current experience; the second is accessing the previous, deep trance experience by utilizing the anchor which you established in the revivification exercise. We're taking Exercise Two and blending it with Exercise One.)

The third step is to ask them to find a time when they were pleasantly surprised with themselves. Once you calibrate and notice they've accessed the experience, then you do what I did with Cindy. Continue using your trance voice and ask, "Where are you?" You're going to do the same thing that you did in the Revivification Exercise (revivify this experience inside the trance that you've already started). The memory you're asking them for is one in which they were pleasantly surprised.

BRANTLEY: Should they be talking?

Yes, they will be talking if they can. They will probably be speaking slowly and literally . . . . . Slowly . . . . All you need is a couple of words so you know where they are. Then give them the suggestion, "You can easily begin to move your mouth only as quickly as you're ready to tell me about the experience where you pleasantly surprised yourself."

By adding this last piece, they are now three levels down in trance. After they tell you about the experience, provide them with a posthypnotic suggestion. In fact, you may want to write this down. This is really fun and this part isn't necessarily verbatim, but you're going to ask them, *"Think of a new ability, a new behavior, or a new feeling, perhaps even a new belief."* Have them consider or think of a new ability, a new behavior, or a new feeling. Remember, what you've done is you've already elicited and anchored a pleasantly surprised experience and a deep trance experience. You've got a word or two for each. Then you ask the person's *unconscious* to decide outside of conscious awareness where *in the next few days, it will pleasantly surprise you.*

(Laughter) At least one unconscious mind liked it. (More laughter.) At least two unconscious minds liked the suggestion.

So the suggestion is: *"Think of a new ability, a new behavior, a new feeling, perhaps even a new belief you'd like to develop. Have your unconscious decide outside of your conscious awareness where, in the next few days, it will pleasantly surprise you."* Now, to really layer it in, we'll add one final posthypnotic suggestion. This is a different one if you want to write it down: *"Open your eyes only as quickly as your unconscious has completed those arrangements . . . Now . . . ."* and that will reorient them.

Demonstration of Layering Pacing Current Experience And Revivification

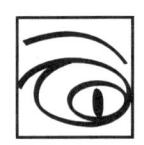

JOHN: So, Cindy, here we are again. (To audience) That's a pace. See how it works? (To Cindy) Here we are again, we're sitting here and you can see those folks over there and one of the things you'll probably start to do . . . . I don't know just when . . . . right . . . (Cindy looks at the trainer) . . . . you can be looking at me, you can be looking at anything really, it doesn't matter. I don't know what you'll be looking at when you stop looking and just sort of **fix your gaze** . . . . . . That's right . . . . (Cindy begins shifting around in the chair.)

*. . . Certainly you can go ahead and make all the adjustments you need to make physically, so that **you're totally comfortable** in a way that works for you. You're probably wondering what this experience will be like. It's good to wonder about experiences such as this because one of the things that's really fun is not knowing just when . . . your eyes will close involuntarily. Hearing the sounds of the room, writing, all the while hearing the sound of my voice. So it's not important whether you're hearing the other things or just hearing my voice.*

You don't have to pay attention to your right arm. You don't have to pay attention to your left arm. You don't have to pay attention to the back of the chair. All you're paying attention to is what I'm saying is the only important thing you need to do . . . . Perhaps you haven't noticed a tendency for those eyes to want to blink. And I don't know when that will be. Not yet. (Eyes blink and once again she shifts in her chair) *. . . . . Or just how much more comfortable you can get and that's right. But it certainly will be interesting once they blink* (eyes blink) *again, when you're paying attention to . . . (eyes blink in an exaggerated way) . . . that's right!*

56   TRAINING TRANCES

>...And how much more attention will you put on your hand before you don't see it except in your mind, **Now** ...... (eyes close).... That's right. With each breath that you take, the deeper you may notice you can go ... **deeper** ...... Because you know as well as I do that you're a great hypnotic subject. You're ..... (Facial muscles go flaccid, chin drops slightly) .... that's right ... you noticed. That's right. It's almost like the time before this one. That's right. When you heard those words. And that **warmth.** That's right. Takes you even deeper and how much more intensely are you experiencing it this time than you did the last? That's right.
>
>...And I don't know just when there was a time in your past.... that you can go deep in your past to find .... when you **pleasantly surprised** yourself with something you did. I don't know that it was a long, long time ago. Perhaps it isn't. It's just one of those experiences that once you did it, you only realized afterwards how good you are ..... That's right ......You didn't know you were going to pleasantly surprise yourself, but you just did. (Cindy begins smiling slowly and nodding cataleptically) .... That's right. The wonderful thing about this state is that you can easily talk to me and remain in this state ... and you can, can you not? . ... So where are you?

CINDY: Speaking.

JOHN: Speaking. And where are you speaking?

CINDY: A conference.

JOHN: A conference. How old are you?

CINDY: Thirty.

JOHN: Thirty .... speaking in front of an audience. That's right. It's wonderful to be surprised like that, isn't it? ..... To feel that good about yourself and your ability .... (pause) .... Who knows what new ability or behavior or maybe feeling, or maybe even belief that you'd like to have in the future .... Something that once you had achieved it, you would feel surprised, pleasantly surprised at yourself in the same way as Cindy there speaking ... ..

> (smiles and nods again) . . . . *That's right.*
>
> *So I'd like you, her unconscious mind, to go ahead and consider where you could create this new behavior, experience, state, or belief . . . where you could produce this outside of her conscious mind, that's right. So that you, her unconscious mind, can surprise her conscious mind and that would be all right . . . . Very good . . . . !*
>
> *So that you can have that same experience of being **pleasantly surprised** just as you are in front of a group, thirty-ish, speaking, all the good feelings you get to take with you . . . . (pause) . . . . and that itself is a **deep experience** in a different way than when you heard . . . . . that's right . . . . **warm** . . . .*
> *. . . So that you can begin to open your eyes only as quickly as your unconscious has completed all of its arrangements . . . So that you can open your eyes and feel refreshed, alert, and awake and open your eyes . . . . . . Great . . . . Give her a hand!*

As you're assisting the person in coming out of trance, you're doing two things. First of all, to the degree you create parallel construction between the beginning and the end of trance, the middle sections will tend to drop out of awareness. We're also chaining the anchors we set as she's coming out of trance. Those states are then chained together to create a powerful resource which is then sandwiched between the original suggestions and the last post-hypnotic suggestion.

What was interesting was that she came out of trance only as quickly as she was complete. There were some things her unconscious mind needed to process before she was going to come the whole way outside and you got to see that. Good job. (To Cindy) **You're a great hypnotic subject.**

SPIKE: I noticed you were using her breathing to create trance. Would you explain that a little further?

The easiest way to develop rapport is to begin speaking on the person's exhale and this will assist them to go into trance. When you want to assist them to come out of trance, watch their breathing and start to speak on their inhale. Give them suggestions and then reorient them. As they begin to rouse from the trance, begin modulating your voice back to a normal conversational level and speak randomly in relation to their breathing.

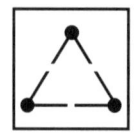

Pacing Current Experience And Revivification Exercise

1. Establish rapport and begin Pacing Current Experience:
   a. use presuppositions of awareness.
   b. lead them from external to internal trance.

2. Fire the anchor for the positive deep trance experience.

3. Elicit and revivify a time when the client was pleasantly surprised:
   a. use Revivification procedure.
   b. it will probably go more slowly because your client is already in trance—you may want to suggest it will be easy for them to speak while remaining in trance.
   c. anchor pleasantly surprised.

4. Suggest: *Think of a new ability, a new behavior, a new feeling, perhaps even a new belief you'd like to develop.* Calibrate and then continue suggesting: *Have your unconscious decide outside of your* conscious awareness where, in the next few days, it will pleasantly *surprise you.*

5. Fire pleasantly surprised anchor.

6. Fire positive deep trance anchor.

7. Provide final posthypnotic suggestion and reorientation: *Open your eyes only as quickly as your unconscious has completed those arrangements . . . . Now!*

Do the exercise

Welcome back.

MEREDITH:
    That induction was awesome.

CHRIS: I liked this because the client does the work and their unconscious will produce the new behavior when it is the most appropriate time for them . . . in their own time . . . and they'll probably forget what you did with them.

That's right, and that's really where it's at. It's not important that they think the suggestion came from the work you did with them; it's okay if they have amnesia. The purpose is for them to pleasantly surprise themselves and in some way improve the quality of their life.

Our job is to put ourselves out of business. (Laughter) Seriously, if we teach people and assist them in removing their blocks so they're in touch with their resources, then they've become integrated, generative beings. That's really what we want for people. We want to fine tune their responses so they can go out and do it on their own. It's not about us, it's about our clients learning to do it for themselves.

By the way, we didn't want to tell you beforehand that we would teach you amnesia, because if we would have, then some of you might have thought, "Oh, gosh, this is really heavy. I'm not sure if I can do this." We thought instead we would do this inductively with you and then you could have your own experience of it. This protocol is one of the main structures for creating amnesia in an ecological way. Some authors refer to these structures as "nested loops" or "multi-embedded metaphors."[11] You assist your partner or client to go down several levels into trance, do the changework at the deepest level of trance, and then come out of trance in the reverse order of the levels you used entering trance. This parallel construction tends to create amnesia.

Up to this point, we've covered two structures to produce a trance state, Revivification and Pacing Current Experience. We should also mention that these approaches extend well beyond the elicitation of trance. Using them will increase the effectiveness of any form of therapy you may do. Understanding the implications of Revivification can be very enlightening even in "nonhypnotic" psychotherapy—if such a thing really exists! (Another great debate!) Remember, a fundamental principle of Revivification is that the asking of detailed questions will tend to install the state associated with the actual memory—asking specific questions about a client's problem will revivify the problem. It may be important to do this in the beginning of a therapy session, because it's usually necessary to bring the problem into the therapy room so that the client can change. However, often excessive time is spent on collecting information which revivifies the problem. Consequently, when the therapist is ready to move on and elicit the outcome or other positive states, the client can't access those states. Why? Because, the retrieval of information is state-dependent. Positive states are not immediately available while the client is inside the problem state. Within the problem state, at best, all the client will be able to do is to redefine the problem state—they'll relate what they had thought about or <u>tried</u> to do about the problem that hasn't worked. If any of these perspectives on the problem would have worked, they wouldn't be seeing you for therapy. Understanding Revivification underscores the importance of calibrating to the client's response to your questions. At times you may ask a client a question which inadvertently and spontaneously elicits a resourceful, positive state for them. Spontaneous states like this that are often the most intense. When you notice this, utilize it. You can either ask more questions about it to further revivify and anchor it, or at the minimum, you may just want to file it away so that you use it later.

Pacing and leading current experience is the cornerstone of all effective therapeutic approaches, as well as for communication in general. **Effective communication is a series of agreements.** Matching and mirroring the client's verbal and nonverbal communication immediately provides for a common starting point. A useful rule of thumb is to only move one lead (or suggestion) beyond the last agreement (pace) with the client. *Be willing* to use whatever verbal or nonverbal responses they communicate to you. This is what makes this approach so much fun. It provides an overall structure of how to proceed with your client, while at the same time it offers lots of room to improvise creatively. Every induction is different. Implementing pacing and leading into your behavior will greatly increase your flexibility in working with a wide variety of clients who may not fit easily into the traditional models of hypnotherapy or psychotherapy.

Next we're going to weave in Conscious-Unconscious Dissociation and formal ideomotor signals. Then we'll be ready for the elicitation of classical hypnotic phenomena, also known as hypnotic skills. What we want to demonstrate to you is the possibility of using hypnosis for more than just "working on your issues." In addition to doing remedial change, you can also make recursive, proactive kinds of changes. That's essentially the design of this training *in trance:* to use each exercise to help you prepare yourself for the next exercise so that you're building recursive loops which will install the process of learning to learn hypnosis . . . . Cogitate on that . . . . for a*while **you learn! NOW . . . . !***

Chapter 4

Dissociating Functions— Communicating Possibilities

Editor's Notes: This chapter highlights the third method for inducing trance which the trainers modeled from Erickson's work: Conscious-Unconscious Dissociation. Elegant demonstrations of this method and ideomotor signaling are both presented.

This "live" demo occurred on Day Two of the training and signaled a shift for the participants. Because the demo subject modeled such enthusiasm and deep rapport with his unconscious mind, he unconsciously assisted the other participants in trusting their unconscious minds more deeply. Their shift was evidenced by the quality of the exercise which followed. In training, the quality of the demonstration determines the quality of the subsequent exercise. Throughout this seminar, there were many shifts similar to this one as the "meta" outcomes for the training occurred. Perhaps the trainers' most singular purpose in doing a training such as this was simply to structure it in a way which would allow the participants to trust their unconscious minds more fully.

For the reader's enjoyment: You may want to have two people read Table 4.1 Features/Functions of The "Two Minds" to you, so you can have a direct experience of Conscious-Unconscious Dissociation.

Conscious-Unconscious Dissociation

The third major structure in Erickson's work for inducing trance is referred to as **Conscious-Unconscious Dissociation.** Either implicitly or explicitly, he used this structure in almost all of his hypnotherapy interviews. He would explain conscious processes as being limited in scope and would then frame the existence of the problem as a limitation of the conscious mind. He may have said something like this to his client: "Yes, you have tried many times to change this particular behavior, and it's not a behavior which the conscious mind can change, and that's why it hasn't changed yet." Erickson viewed the unconscious as a source of wisdom, so he would always suggest that the solution to the problem was to be found in the unconscious mind. He defined the conscious mind as limited and the unconscious as unlimited. Creating this contrast between the "two minds" allowed him to explain almost any problem as a function of the conscious mind and the solution as a function of the unconscious mind. One of his most famous quotes is, "Your patients will be your patients because they are out of rapport with their unconscious mind."[1] Essentially he was saying if a problem exists, it's because we're not accessing (or in rapport with) our unconscious, unlimited resources.

This metaphor of the "two minds" can be quite generative in the changes it produces. Not only does it provide a basis for creating solutions, it recognizes possibilities and connections well beyond the resolution of the problem itself. The functions of the unconscious mind are far more versatile and diverse than the mere remediation of problems. Examples of functions which may expand spontaneously when one is in rapport with one's unconscious are creativity, learning to learn, and redefining the self. The induction itself can be easily developed and expanded to incorporate much of the research done since the 1970s on hemispheric specialization,[2] holographic models of memory,[3] and psychoneuroimmunology[4,5] which substantiate the unlimited potential of the unconscious mind. The model ought to be adjusted and expanded to the client's presenting problem and his or her model of the world. Conscious-Unconscious Dissociation may also be used as a therapeutic intervention and is discussed in Chapter Seven.

In this section, we're focusing on the effectiveness of Conscious-Unconscious Dissociation as a trance induction. It's a valuable technique for working with someone who's particularly intellectual or who requires cognitive education about the roles of the conscious and unconscious minds. Doing cognitive education is fun because we can have a "nice, educational" conversation while we're also observing the effect the dissociation is having on the client. We're only educating them at this point, not doing a formal trance induction! That's classic Erickson!

Here are some of the concepts associated with the conscious mind and the unconscious mind which you can use to create dissociation. You could literally read down the list on page 66 as you do your trance induction. Before we share the full conscious explanation of this process, we'd like you to experience it unconsciously first.

JOHN: Your conscious mind can be aware of seven ± two chunks of information and your conscious mind can pay attention to whatever is going on at the time.

JULIE: While your unconscious mind knows everything else.

JOHN: Your conscious mind tends to think in a sequential way, because it thinks one thing has to go after another.

JULIE: And your unconscious deals in simultaneity; it has the possibility of dealing with everything simultaneously.

JOHN: Your conscious mind is logical.

JULIE: Your unconscious mind is intuitive and it associates new learnings easily.

JOHN: Your conscious mind tends to think in terms of cause and effect; it's linear. It says this makes that happen: one thing after another in the same way so that it is sequential and logical.

JULIE: Your unconscious mind knows everything is a cybernetic loop, that one thing merely influences the other, not one thing causes the other. Your unconscious mind knows it's a cybernetic system.

JOHN: Your conscious mind is constantly asking, why is this true? Why is this the way that it is?

JULIE: Your unconscious mind knows why.

JOHN: The conscious mind generally is the part of you which does the thinking. All the regular thinking, the intellectual thinking which you engage in during the course of the day.

JULIE: Which makes it easier for your unconscious to do all your feeling.

JOHN: Your conscious mind is generally equated with your waking state.

JULIE: And your unconscious with your sleeping and dreaming state.

JOHN: Consciously, you can voluntarily move parts of your body.

JULIE: Yet it's your unconscious which moves your body involuntarily.

JOHN: Consciously, you can be aware only of what is happening right now.

JULIE: Yet your unconscious is the storehouse of all your memories.

JOHN: Conscious mind tries to understand problems. It thinks that by understanding problems, it won't have the problem.

JULIE: If only it would allow the unconscious mind which does know the solution to present you with the solution, then your conscious mind can . . .

JOHN: Direct the outcome. Your conscious mind can decide what it wants all the rest of you to do.

JULIE: While your unconscious mind expedites the outcome.

JOHN: Conscious mind is deliberate.

JULIE: Unconscious is automatic.

JOHN: Conscious mind is verbal.

JULIE: Unconscious is nonverbal.

JOHN: Conscious mind is analytical.

JULIE: Unconscious mind is able to synthesize things.

JOHN: Conscious mind is most effective when tending to information that's occurring.

JULIE: While the unconscious mind records all the information to which the conscious mind has attended.

JOHN: So the conscious mind has a limited focus.

JULIE: And the unconscious mind has an unlimited expansive focus.

JOHN: The conscious mind is the domain of your cognitive learnings and understandings.

Dissociating Functions—Communicating Possibilities

JULIE: And the unconscious mind is the domain of all your experiential learnings.

JOHN: Notice what that does. How many of you experienced a feeling of something spreading apart or expanding? What we did was very minimal because we virtually read down the list and added only a few words. In actual practice, you may not even need to use the whole list. You can be selective. There are a number of other nuances we'll be adding which will make this far more effective than what you've just experienced. Additionally, you can combine this particular approach with Pacing Current Experience . . . So, as you're sitting here, you can pay attention to me consciously . . .

JULIE: And your conscious mind, that logical part, can wonder what this is really all about.

JOHN: While your unconscious mind can really be getting to grips with the source of why you're here.

JULIE: And while your unconscious is doing that, your conscious mind on some level may still be asking why, why would we be doing any of this in the first place?

JOHN: And consciously you can consider what your outcome is. Consciously you can even make a picture of you at the end of the training.

JULIE: You can think about it consciously for as long as you like.

JOHN: Because it's your unconscious mind that will go back through your history and find all the resourceful experiences you need to combine in various ways that will make that outcome happen.

JULIE: And you'll know you've had that outcome when your unconscious signals you with the right feeling.

JOHN: But that's not nearly as important as being consciously aware of what's being said right now each time your eyes blink.

JULIE: And for some of you your eyes blink automatically.

JOHN: Unconsciously.

Table 4.1
FEATURES/FUNCTIONS OF THE "TWO MINDS"

Conscious ——————— Unconscious

Dissociation

Conscious	Unconscious
7 ± 2 chunks	everything else
sequential	simultaneous
logical	intuitive, associational
linear	cybernetic
asks "why"	knows why
thinking	feeling
waking	sleeping, dreaming
voluntary movements	involuntary movements
aware of now	storehouse of all memories
tries to understand problem	knows solution
directs outcome	expedites outcome
deliberate	automatic
verbal	nonverbal
analytical	synthetic
attends to information	attends/records information
limited focus	unlimited, expansive
cognitive learnings	experiential learnings

Dr. Erickson might start an induction by saying, "Your conscious mind can just go ahead and sit there and pay attention to that spot on the wall, or listen to the sound of my voice, because I'm not interested in talking to your conscious mind. I'm interested in talking to your unconscious mind." So he was beginning even in the first sentence to separate the two minds, all the while blending in the client's current experience.

Initially when you're Pacing Current Experience, you will want to attribute to the unconscious mind any automatic behavior which the client displays. Eye blinking, swallowing, and breathing, for example, are labelled as unconscious occurrences. Your conscious mind doesn't usually know when *your eyes are going to blink* next because the *unconscious mind will blink those eyes.* (Wait until eyes blink.) That's right . . . So your conscious mind can only wonder just when those eyes are going to . . . (Say "blink" this time at the same time you see the eyes blink). All that it can do is wait for *your unconscious to go ahead and make them blink.* Have you ever been driving down a road with the windows open, or maybe you're riding your bike, and there's a bug coming toward you and you don't see it with your conscious mind, but *your unconscious mind makes those eyes close* (snap) *that fast, reflexively?* You know what it feels like when your eyes close reflexively, don't you? That's right, not yet though. Because there's still a lot more you can see out here (hear).What I'm saying is important for you to understand, consciously as well.

This process is called Dissociation—dissociating the conscious mind from the unconscious mind and vice versa. We create boundaries around each function of the mind and then juxtapose them. Creating this split (yet simultaneous) awareness of two separate minds will produce trance. It's very effective in creating trance because most people don't have this split awareness in their normal, everyday consciousness. When the two minds are dissociated from one another, an altered state—i.e., trance—occurs which is different from their normal, waking state.

General Steps For Conscious-Unconscious Dissociation

Remember, you always begin by matching and mirroring your partner or client and lead them into trance by modeling it for them. You'll use the Features/Functions of the "Two Minds" (Table 4.1, page 66) and induce a trance by Pacing Current Experience. Now, if some of you feel inclined to assist the person in also revivifying an experience, we can't stop you, okay? Try as you might to hold yourself back, *you can go ahead* and try to hold yourself back from not injecting a *revivification experience* into it. And we're not asking you to actually *go ahead and do it*. We're really only doing Conscious-Unconscious Dissociation, but you never know consciously what happens when you're in trance until it does!

Establishing "Yes" And "No" Signals With The Unconscious Mind

Next, you're going to establish formal "yes/no" signals with your partner's unconscious mind. This is also known as "ideomotor signaling." There are many ways you can do this. You've seen people in conversation and you know when they're agreeing with one another because they may be nodding their heads "yes." (Trainers are nodding heads very subtly and slowly.) You know when they're disagreeing because they may begin to shake their heads ever so slightly (trainers model subtly) while you're speaking to them . . . just in a normal conversation

You can just as easily signal with your hands. How many of you remember what you did in school if you needed something? What did you always have to do first? That's right, raise your hand. You would raise your hand if you wanted to communicate "Yes, I want to" or "Yes, I know the answer." After the teacher responded to you, then you knew it was time to put your hand down. If the teacher was asking a question to which you didn't yet know the answer, you knew to keep your hand down. You also knew to keep your hand down if the teacher wanted volunteers and you didn't want to participate.

Sometimes people like to signal in a more formal way . . . you've probably experienced this . . . in restaurants . . . a nice restaurant . . . when you want to signal the server, "Yes, I want something," you raise your finger politely . . Now, some people may raise their entire hand but when you're at a service-oriented restaurant where you're always attended to, there's no need to say a word, just a finger or even a look will do and you understand that, do you not?

This is very similar to how Erickson would set up unconscious signals with his clients' unconscious minds. He'd use indirect suggestion as we did above, to create associations rather than directly telling the client to lift one finger for a "yes" and another finger for a "no." The associations will activate neural networks which will potentiate fine motor movements. If you're going to use direct suggestion later, using indirect suggestion first will increase the client's response potential. By using indirect suggestion (association), you activate the neural networks (memories) before you give a direct suggestion indicating a particular response. If you do this, the client may actually display the unconscious behavior before you ever formally request it. If they don't, it's still okay because at the least you've opened up the neural pathways, thereby increasing receptivity to the actual direct suggestion when it is provided.

Another method which is more direct and yet very naturalistic is the beginning of the Six-Step Reframe procedure[6] which was modeled from Erickson's work. In this protocol you ask, *"Is your unconscious mind willing to communicate?"* (Usually you would ask, "Is your unconscious mind willing to communicate to you consciously?" if you wanted conscious awareness.) You then calibrate to your client's minimal cues. Once you notice the signal, you ask the unconscious to *intensify that response for a "yes" signal* (calibrate) and then ask it to *diminish the intensity of the response (or ask for an opposing response) to signal a "no" response.* This has traditionally been done with the client's conscious participation as they would verbalize which internal response they noticed. If you're doing it this way, you ought to have some way other than their verbal report to calibrate to their response. It's generally easier to do it without their verbal report because there's less chance of conscious editing and filtering. Also if they're in a deep trance, they'll probably have to come out to some extent to respond verbally.

Leslie LeCron, a well-known psychologist who specializes in hypnosis, is really the person who popularized the use of finger signals.[7] He frequently used direct suggestion and would say to the client, "The forefinger of your right hand will lift for a 'yes' and the forefinger of your left hand will lift for a 'no.' You can lift the little finger of your right hand for 'I don't know' and the little finger of your left hand for 'I don't want to tell.'"

When your client is in a comfortable trance, that's when you'll establish "yes" and "no" signals. Suggest the following: *"Your unconscious mind can always communicate this way in trance so its intentions can be recognized and respected. And does your unconscious mind understand that?"* Then what are you going to wait for? A signal. If you receive a "no" response, it has communicated to you. Respect its wishes and ask what its purpose is in giving the "no" response. Asking for the purpose is also known as "chunking up" to a higher logical level of abstraction.

A useful qualifying suggestion is to ask for a response with *"honest" unconscious movements.* "Honest" is an indication that you want a response directly from the unconscious mind. Unconscious movements will tend to be short, jerky movements, rather than quick, smooth movements. For some folks who haven't done this before, it might take as long as two or three minutes for them to develop a full finger response. Other people will do it rather quickly.

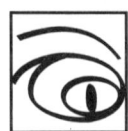

Demonstration of Conscious-Unconscious Dissociation With Ideomotor Signals

JULIE: Who's our subject today? Brantley—all right, come on up. So you're up here because you want to go in trance, right?

BRANTLEY: I'm already in trance.

JULIE: You *are* in a trance. So, let me ask you, is it okay if I look at them while I sometimes talk to you?

BRANTLEY: Yes.

JULIE: And *you understand* that I'm still here with you even though I'm looking at them, over there?

BRANTLEY: Uh huh.

JULIE: Thank you. So, is it your conscious mind that's in a trance, right now, or is it your unconscious mind that's entrancing your conscious mind to *go into that trance, now?*

BRANTLEY: They're kind of together.

JULIE: Ah. Does your conscious mind, Brantley, like to play with your unconscious?

BRANTLEY: This time.

JULIE: And how does your unconscious like it when it has a playmate?

BRANTLEY: Great.

JULIE: Good, very good. So your conscious mind . . . that's right . . .

JULIE: that's right . . . can just ease more fully into paying attention to what I'm saying. I'd like to invite your conscious mind (spoken in a conversational voice) to clearly listen to everything and to fully experience everything that happens, including the honking of a horn outside this room, as *your unconscious mind* (spoken in a trance voice) *learns everything it wants to about the hypnotic relationship.* (Conscious-Unconscious Dissociation has begun.)

Now I'd like to ask your unconscious, is that hypnotic relationship the one between your conscious and *you're unconscious,* or is it the hypnotic relationship between the subject and the operator? I'll leave it to your conscious mind to think it knows the answer, and your unconscious mind to experience the answer . . . so as you fully focus right there (fixation of attention) . . . where your eye . . that's right . . . letting your conscious mind not know fully when you're blinking . . . that's right . . . letting your unconscious mind . . . that's right . . . blink when it does, your conscious mind can only wonder, Brantley, when you will *close your eyes* (eyes close) . . . very good . . . as your unconscious mind knows thoroughly the exact plan that it has for you today . . .

Otherwise, *your unconscious* would have not invited you, its conscious mind, to *participate fully* by coming up and entering into trance . . . very good. Now, your conscious mind can notice the slight fluttering of those eyelids (eyes are closed and fluttering rapidly), and *I'd like to congratulate the unconscious for demonstrating* that (unconscious signals) to the group. They really do like to see great hypnotic subjects, and that little flickering of the eyes means that *you're going into the next level of the trance* . . . excellent! And your breathing confirms that to your conscious mind (deep breath, shifted much lower into the abdomen).

Now, I don't know what your conscious mind is doing in there to play with your unconscious mind. I do know that *your unconscious knows,* and I know perhaps your conscious is beginning to know what things it can do to play with your unconscious mind. I'd just like to invite them to *go right ahead and play,* and I'm not even sure if playing is a conscious activity or an unconscious activity. I just *know that playing is fun,* and I think you should *play as much as you want,* both consciously and *unconsciously.*

JULIE: Because in the spirit of play, *I'd like to invite your **unconscious mind**, as a great hypnotic subject, to **communicate with us**. So, in a moment I am going to just ask you to answer by signaling with your head a slight nod, an honest, unconscious, **slow nod for a "Yes"**... nice and slow ... whenever you're ready. Now I'd like to ask your unconscious mind when you do nod your head, "yes."* (Head nods cataleptically.) *That's right, very good ... excellent.*

Now, I'd like to let your conscious mind know that it's doing a most excellent job in maintaining rapport with the unconscious mind, and that means the learnings you are having as a demo subject .. because you know who learns the most, in an exercise like this? .. <u>is</u> the demo subject. So the learnings that you're grasping here represent a new bridge which is being built between your conscious and you're unconscious ... mind ... to take you deeper ... is a foundation that can last for a long, long, long time. And you understand what that means, do you not? (Head nods cataleptically again) *... That's right ... all honest unconscious head nods.*

*Excellent ... and I see that your conscious and unconscious thoroughly understand the hypnotic relationship that is occurring here, right now. I'd like to let both of those minds know that I'm holding a very favorable internal representation, as well as external, verbal representation to the students observing you about what a great ... not only hypnotic subject you are ... but what great rapport is existing on a deeper and deeper level between your two minds. And as a demonstration of that, if you would be kind enough just to play and show us an honest, **unconscious headshake from left to right, right to left**, back and forth, forth and back, whichever way you want to do it, a little headshake back and forth, that we will know for Brantley **means "no"**... excellent ... that's right ...* (head shakes back and forth very slowly) *Very, very good ... I see that you understand not only what I said and not only what your conscious and unconscious have communicated to one another .. but that you fully understand their internal representation of you as you're sitting there learning how to lead great hypnotic subjects. Watch "me"* (referring to Brantley) *... that's right ... you understand ... very good ... very good ... We all need someone in our lives to show us the way. You know that, and you know what that means to you and your life. I know what it meant to me and my life. And I thank your unconscious and conscious for showing us how to do it.*

JULIE: *Now, as a further demonstration, if you would be kind enough to signal them, out there, the participants in this room, learning to* **have rapport** *between their conscious and unconscious mind in a way that you have modeled for us here today. Would you be kind enough to* **lift your right forefinger, your right index finger for a "yes" and your left for a "no"?** (Trainer demonstrates direct suggestion for ideomotor signals due to depth of trance.) *And you can wait to do that until I ask you a question. When I ask you a question, you can lift your right forefinger for a "yes"* . . . (slight lifting movement of right forefinger). *That's right . . . and your left forefinger for a "no." Does your unconscious mind and your conscious mind understand my directions?* (Brantley signals with right forefinger) *. . . very good . . . excellent . . . perfect . . . a good honest, unconscious response. And are you ready to come out of the trance yet? . . .* (right forefinger raises) *Yes . . . you are? . . . very good . . excellent.*

Are you awake now Brantley? Tell us, are you awake now? (left finger raises slightly) *that's good . . . excellent . . . See, because you and I are not only communicating . . . not only for you . . . and not only for the people in the room . . . we're communicating in this way for other relationships in your life where the increased rapport between your conscious and unconscious mind will manifest. Frankly, I don't know who that may be and neither does your conscious mind, yet. All that I am concerned about is that you've learned, as well as taught us what honest, unconscious trance movements look like. And for that I* **really appreciate your unconscious,** *and I do also really appreciate your conscious mind. You understand that, do you not? . . . And you can say "no" if you do not . . .* (Right finger moves cataleptically.) *Good . . . very good.*

So, what I'd like to suggest . . . that's right . . . loosen it up . . . that's right . . . what I'd like to suggest to your unconscious mind is that you have the ability to always communicate your intentions through your nonverbal gestures with the congruent participation of your conscious and unconscious minds. So that your intentions, Brantley, can always be respected by whoever it is that you come in contact with, as well as you, yourself, respecting your own intentions. (Trainer begins to gradually speak in a more conversational tone, tempo, and volume.) *So, since you are ready to come out of trance, you can certainly . . . only as you* **awaken fully** *. . . that's right . . . and to the degree that you* **have a growing sense of appreciation for you,** *his unconscious mind.* (Brantley takes a minute or two to reorient.)

JULIE: You were magnificent . . . ! (To audience.) Now, we're at a choice point: it's sometimes quite nice to validate the client's experience for them. One way to do that is to process the experience a bit. I'll ask him if he wants to, and if he does want to say a few words, it will be verification to him more than it will provide information for us. If he prefers to stay in silence, that will be fine, too.

(To Brantley) Is there anything that you'd like to share with us about your experience, that you'd like to mention to us?

BRANTLEY:
Well, it was pretty weird, and it was pretty wonderful, too. It was as if you could be in two places at the same time [excellent confirmation of the Conscious-Unconscious Dissociation] and know it. It was kind of like that . . . and it was real weird, because my conscious mind was busy doing seven plus or minus . . . keeping track of whatever, doing everything that my unconscious mind was telling it to do. It was pretty neat.

I've also been thinking about how exciting it is whenever my conscious and my unconscious mind are congruent. So before the induction, I suggested to myself that it would be okay to go into trance in a different way than I usually do . . . so that my unconscious mind and my conscious mind would be able to work together. I thought it would be really neat if they did that and enjoy it as they did it.

JULIE: And they did, didn't they?

BRANTLEY:
Yeah, they really did.

JULIE: Great job . . . one of the best parts of this demo is the clarity of Brantley's unconscious movements. His signals were so clear and honest, they would have been an excellent example for a training video. So—anything else?

BRANTLEY:
No, I don't think so.

JULIE: That's right, you don't <u>think</u> so! Thanks, Brantley . . . Let's give him a hand.

BRANTLEY:
> Thank you.

> **Conscious-Unconscious Dissociation With Ideomotor Signaling Exercise**
>
> 1. Establish rapport. Incorporate the client's current experience while using Conscious-Unconscious Dissociation. Some additional nuances, if you like to add them:
>   a. tonal anchors for conscious and unconscious.
>   b. linkage words: start with simple conjunctives and progress to causative verbs.
>   c. as trance progresses, proportionately more time should be spent talking to the unconscious rather than the conscious. (Reverse this coming out of trance.)
>
> 2. Deepen the trance.
>
> 3. Establish "yes" and "no" signals.
>
> 4. Posthypnotic suggestion:
>   "Your unconscious mind can always communicate this way in trance so it's intentions can be recognized and respected. And does your unconscious mind understand that?" Calibrate.
>
> 5. Reorient.

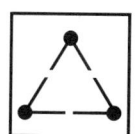

Do the exercise

Discussion

Welcome back.

BRANTLEY:
> How often do people signal "yes" in one way, for example using their finger, then use a different activity to signal "no"? While my partner was doing "yes," she was doing a head nod. But when she did "no," there was very little signal except for her facial expression.

That's a good question. One of the things which can happen with some people is you'll ask for a "yes" response, and you'll get a fairly obvious "yes" response. Then you ask for a "no" response, and sometimes you'll just get an absence of a "yes" response. That can happen. The way to set that up so you're more likely to have something different is to ask the unconscious mind "to provide an opposing signal," or words to that effect. So for most people an opposing signal to a "yes" wouldn't be keeping their head still, it would be shaking it "no." Generally speaking, if it's lifting the right forefinger for a "yes," most of the time it will interpret "an opposing signal" as meaning it will lift the left forefinger for a "no." That's another way of doing it.

As mentioned earlier, another way of doing it is by asking the unconscious to intensify the signal for a "yes" and diminish it for a "no." That works well, too. In my opinion, that takes more calibration skill and a little more finesse. The finger signals are really much easier; they're obvious. After establishing clear finger signals, you'll know fairly quickly if things aren't proceeding. You'll get "no" responses and you'll know that you're not misreading the situation. So, generally, if you ask for an opposing stimulus or response, that will provide you with a different response.

Sometimes just establishing signals can have profound effects, because it really fosters increasing rapport between the conscious and unconscious minds. I worked with a young man who was an interesting referral. His family referred him to me, and he had so many big issues in his life that I didn't have a clue about where to start. To top it off, he only wanted to come for a one-hour session, and that was it. After about fifteen minutes or so, we got it narrowed down to of all things, quitting smoking, which is not something I would do in an hour without any preparation. I guess I was feeling frisky that day so I decided, what the heck, I might as well see what we could do.

I couldn't really help him to be congruent about wanting to quit smoking, but he thought that he ought to stop it. I tried to do some of the more obvious NLP interventions, and they went nowhere. Nothing was happening. With about ten minutes left in the session, I had him put his hands on his legs and asked him to move one finger for a "yes" and another for a "no." He experienced the responses and was really impressed with himself. He was into paranormal phenomena, so I said, "This will really help you because *you'll have increased communication with your unconscious mind.*" All I did was ask his unconscious mind the question, "Does your unconscious mind love you?" That was it, that's all we did. He called up a week later to tell me he had totally quit smoking. It was the most miraculous thing that ever happened to him, and I had been thinking I had no idea what I did.

I've seen both of his parents at different points for therapy, and they said he's doing excellently. He had opened his own business, was in a steady relationship and had also stopped drinking. He did all this and I thought—just with finger signals? Who knows? I don't want to suggest that by just setting up finger signals people will change, just because they have an enhanced rapport with their unconscious mind. That's probably more than you ought to expect. What I am suggesting, though, is that it is a real beginning to help a person align their conscious mind with their unconscious mind, so that they have a better way of understanding their unconscious responses. The presence of ideomotor responses provides them with a convincer, or an external way of validating that they are actually communicating with their unconscious mind.

ROBERT:
    Do you prefer to have the unconscious make the decision about the actual ideomotor responses which it is going to use?

That depends. You want to be comfortable doing it with either direct or indirect suggestion. In indirect suggestion, we'll set up a double bind—like we don't know which finger of which hand is going to want to lift first for a "yes" response. In direct suggestion, we'll instruct them in which finger to use when. One variable to consider is how well trained your client is. You can invite the unconscious mind to lift whatever finger it would like to lift to signal a "yes." If they are not in rapport with their unconscious, they may sit there for five minutes and not lift anything. You may want to educate them by saying, "I'd like you to go ahead and lift your left finger for a 'no,' and your right finger for a 'yes.'" Then reach over and pick up their finger while you're suggesting, "This finger can lift for a 'yes.'" Do the same for "no." Then ask, "Does your unconscious mind understand?" It's easier to have them practice with your assistance rather than waiting for them to respond. If they're a completely untrained subject, you might want to assist in the beginning.

    Another variable to consider is the depth of their trance. Remember, the deeper the trance, the more you want to use direct suggestion. If the person is in a very deep trance, you may save yourself a lot of time by just suggesting which finger should be lifted for "yes" and which for "no." If they're in a lighter trance and you're not doing a long deepening process, then you may want to use examples which are done by implication and presupposition. Being more indirect is probably going to be your better way to go. If you get the signals at that point, fine. If not, you can also directly suggest the responses you want later on.

    Also, some schools of hypnosis prefer to have the client choose, while others prefer to have the hypnotherapist choose. Rather than being dogmatic about which way is the right way, it's more important to trust your intuition, or unconscious mind, and use the way which it knows is best at the particular time. Again, it's important for us to have the flexibility to go either or both ways, depending on our client's responses.

LEE: I noticed that you had arranged two different ways for Brantley's unconscious mind to signal "yes" and "no." Should we set up more than one way? Also, if the client is reclining or lying down, head nods may not work that well.

Generally, when you're working with clients, one is certainly sufficient. Since he was such a great subject, I wanted to show you as many examples as I possibly could of honest, unconscious movement. His movements were very pure and very clear. Doing more than one was just to demonstrate to you what the head nod and the head shake would look like, as well as what the finger signals would look like, so you would have examples of both. In a real life situation, I would have only done one as long as it produced the results.

DON: Speaking of unconscious signals, what if your client falls asleep while they're in trance?

If your client's lying on the floor, and he's snoring, he's not in trance! You have received, however, an unconscious signal, just not the one you were expecting. Clients may transition from trance to physiological sleep. To double-check if they are really asleep or not, calibrate to them, provide some suggestions, and notice if they follow you. If they follow the suggestions, you can proceed because they are in a deep trance and just appear to be sleeping. If they're actually asleep, it's best to gently wake them in some way, because they're not going to get much value from the suggestions. Remember when we thought it was a good idea to listen to foreign language tapes while sleeping, so you would learn to speak Spanish, French, etc.? Some dream! If only it would have worked! We now know we need sleep for incorporation and integration.[8] Trying to add and encode new information at this stage can interrupt these naturally occurring processes.

So, if your client falls asleep, it may be a communication to you that you've temporarily lost rapport. To regain rapport, you can begin crossover mirroring. For example, match your words to their breathing and give them a suggestion that in a moment you will gently tap them on their hand, and that will remind them to pay attention to what is important. Continue this until you regain contact with them. Meanwhile *both of you can rest assured* sleep has its own benefits. Because while you sleep *you can dream*, and dreams can have lasting, profound, beneficial, *transforming* effects that can stay with you for the rest of *your life*. Is that an <u>in</u>bedded suggestion? Nod really. So that you, too, can rest assured you're one at the deepest levels of integration.

And when *you wake up*, for some funny reason you may discover a growing interest in catalepsy that won't be satisfied until you . . . That's right!

Chapter 5

Catalepsy: Giving Your Trancework A Healing Lift

Editor's Notes: To assist the participants and readers, this training is sequenced in the same order as the hypnotic interview. Preframing or some type of setup is the first step. Next, an induction occurs to elicit trance. Then, if appropriate, a hypnotic phenomenon is selected to deepen trance or to set up the changework section. The trainers have covered the first two steps in Chapters One through Four and are now ready to explore hypnotic phenomena. Because the trainers value catalepsy so highly, it is the subject of this entire chapter.

Three excellent inductions to induce catalepsy are included, all with graphic demonstrations, including one with a subject who is unsure of her trance abilities. The reader may be surprised at how easy these inductions are to initiate. After reading this chapter, and with a little practice, the reader ought to be able to utilize and demonstrate these techniques easily. The trainers' favorite induction for catalepsy is the simplest. It relies upon a hypnotic response which everyone has and begins with, "If we were meeting for the first time I would say, 'Hi, my name is J....'" Several other models to elicit catalepsy are also explored.

The chapter concludes with a valuable discussion about the implications of catalepsy for healing.

Now that you understand the structure of Erickson's trance inductions, the next area to consider is that of Hypnotic Phenomena. Hypnotic phenomena, or hypnotic skills, demonstrate to the conscious mind the countless possibilities available within the hypnotic or trance state. This section will be devoted to one of the foremost examples of hypnotic phenomena: catalepsy. In our opinion, catalepsy is one of the "classics" in the field. It was first described by Charcot in 1882[1] and its use continues today. Catalepsy is respected as a valuable and versatile hypnotic tool. Erickson discusses its use as a form of ideomotor signaling for inducing trance.[2] Based upon Erickson's work and our clinical experience, we have observed that when catalepsy is developed as a skill, it becomes an obvious example of gaining control over involuntary, physiological responses. Therefore, we have utilized it as one way to access the body's deeper "intelligence" in assisting clients in the healing "crisis" to communicate with their unconscious minds.

Catalepsy is a physiological condition where balanced tonicity exists between the agonist and antagonist muscles.[3] An example is arm levitation. In hypnosis, if arm levitation is suggested and catalepsy occurs, it will feel as if your arm is lifting itself involuntarily. In the trance state and with the acceptance of the suggestions, your unconscious mind will be moving it for you. During catalepsy, the kinesthetics and the proprioceptive senses are quite different from those you experience when you lift your arm voluntarily. This seems to be because the balance between flexion and extension is different from the balance for voluntary responses.

(Trainer demonstrates with his arm while in an autohypnotic trance.)

(To audience.) As my arm moves up, notice it moves relatively slowly, in small jerky movements, almost as if it's being lifted by a winch. If you look at my fingers now, they're somewhat extended, pretty firm and my whole hand is beginning to become cataleptic. If the suggestion was given that my arm should remain suspended, someone could try to push it up or down and it would stay exactly where it is, because it's "frozen" in the cataleptic state.

When catalepsy develops, the body part which is affected manifests "waxy flexibility." Waxy flexibility is a well-known psychiatric term describing catatonia.[4] Catatonic schizophrenics are in a state of total catalepsy most of the time. They're the ones that if you put their arm out like this (arm outstretched at shoulder height to demonstrate catalepsy) and come back two hours later, they're still in the exact same position. However, like many other types of behavior, processes which appear dysfunctional in one context can be extraordinarily resourceful in another. Such is catalepsy. As we go on, you'll see that catalepsy may be used to induce trance, deepen trance, initiate analgesia and anesthesia, create partial dissociation, and provide ideomotor signaling. It's inherent value is that it serves as a "convincer" for the conscious mind and indicates that something out of the ordinary is occurring. It is a compelling metaphor of accomplishing mind/body unity (literally, "yoga" i.e. "union") along with all the other possibilities which researchers are now discovering about the innate healing intelligence of the body.[5,6] As Erickson explained, "Your body is a lot wiser than you are."[7]

Usually you'll begin by Pacing Current Experience while creating Conscious-Unconscious Dissociation at the beginning in the induction phase. If you're interested in inducing a deeper trance, you might add other methods during the induction phase like Revivification, counting, and so on. Always bear in mind that most effective inductions are not this linear, but this gives you a way to initially structure your thinking.

Once you have some indication that your client is in a satisfactory trance, you may want to introduce other hypnotic phenomena which will facilitate the changework you're doing. Arm catalepsy can be paired with suggestions while you're doing the changework. It is an effective ideomotor gauge for how well and how quickly the changework is proceeding. For example, you can suggest that the arm begins to go down only as fast as the unconscious mind can incorporate the new learnings. Erickson used catalepsy this way.

When utilizing catalepsy, you have two primary choices. You may decide to induce trance first and then suggest arm levitation, or you may decide to incorporate catalepsy as part of the initial trance induction itself. One possible drawback to the first method is that the client may go so deeply into trance before you do the arm levitation that it may take awhile for them to lift their hand from their lap. Both ways are useful and it's worthwhile to become confident with each of them—you'll have your own experience of the difference between the methods as well as maximum flexibility when you work with clients.

We'll demonstrate a number of different inductions to produce arm catalepsy for you in this section. Who wants to have an experience of it now?

Demonstration of Surprise Handshake Induction With Catalepsy

Trainer: Dan? We'll start with Dan. (Dan is seated in the front row directly in front of the trainer. He has raised his hand and as soon as the trainer made eye contact with him Dan moved forward slightly in his chair, an excellent unconscious indication of his desire to be a demonstration subject. The trainer then moves toward Dan and gestures to stand up and approach the trainer. Dan does this: again, another example of nonverbal communication and rapport. The trainer now offers his right hand, beginning a handshake. As soon as Dan extends his right hand, the trainer pulls his own hand away slightly and uses his left hand to lightly grasp Dan's right wrist and move it to a distance of about eighteen inches from Dan's face.)

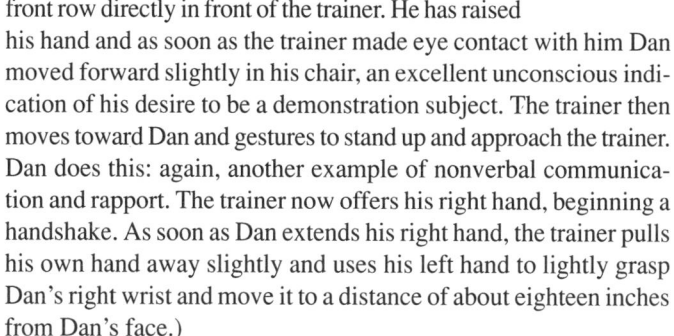

That's right . . . . (Spoken very quickly, in command tonality) . . just look at that hand, as you watch that hand move toward you (trainer is moving Dan's right hand slightly toward Dan's face while trainer's right hand is pointing to Dan's right hand).... you notice the changing focus of your eyes, and as you do, notice the tendency for your *eyes to close* .... (Simultaneously with the phrase, "eyes to close" the trainer moves his right hand from its pointing position downward and away from Dan's focus, so that Dan's eyes follow the trainer's hand.)

[Try this yourself. If you pass your hand downward from eye level, keeping your head still, your eyelids will naturally drop as you follow the hand.]

... As you notice that hand is getting closer and closer to your face (by now Dan's eyes are closed and his hand is moving cataleptically toward his face), that's right, closer and closer, (trainer's voice softens and slows) ..... *until you just allow it to happen ... all the way ... down ... that's right ... all the way down ... while that hand just remains totally fixed ... right there ... that's right ... right there on that shelf ... notice how comfortable it can be right there ... on that shelf ... that's right ... you notice that your entire body can just remain totally fixed and comfortable in that way.* (Dan's entire body is now cataleptic.)

..... *And I'd like to suggest to your unconscious that you are learning ... you are learning how to control involuntary responses, voluntarily, by making that connection with your unconscious. Now, I know and you know too that there is a matter that you have been consciously wanting to deal with ... that's right, I'd like to suggest that through just this experience you can begin to make certain inroads to the unconscious ... realizing that you can communicate with it ... and you can give it the kind of suggestions so that it realizes when it's appropriate to do what it does .... and when it's inappropriate ... that's right ... and your conscious mind doesn't have to necessarily understand fully ... these instructions ... that's right ... but it can allow your unconscious mind to begin to work with that particular issue, not necessarily now, but as you sleep tonight, you can have a number of dreams that will allow you, at the unconscious level, to bring together those resources necessary in order for everything to be whole and healthy the way that you would like. So that you can really begin to notice that change can happen in a clearly spontaneous way ... to your surprise ... that's right ... and I'd like in a moment for your unconscious mind to just let me know once it has completed making those*

*arrangements for later . . . that's right . . . a signal will do . . . . . .
. . . . (Dan nods head) . . . . . that's right . . . once you're complete
. . . very good . . . !*

(Trainer resumes the handshake that had been interrupted and returns to a conversational voice.) So, how are you doing? It is good to see you. It's been awhile. A couple of years since the last time. (Going back to the conversation the trainer began with the handshake induction will increase amnesia for the trance induction.) Good job!

Discussion

The type of induction which I just did with Dan looks dramatic, but I've only done it for demonstration purposes at seminars. It is a surprise induction, so I don't do this when I meet a person for the first time. Erickson did, however. It even came to the point where people didn't want to shake his hand at conferences because they knew what he was going to do.

We're going to show you another pattern which would be more appropriate to do in your office. The key ingredient to any successful handshake induction is interrupting the automatic motor program associated with handshaking. It's common in our culture that when you offer your hand to another person, they're going to shake it. It's unusual for one person to offer their hand and the other person not to follow through by doing the same. When you interrupt this pattern, most people's conscious activity is temporarily suspended. As they search for meaning in your actions, they enter transderivational search (TDS) or trance. They're literally in downtime awaiting the next cue from the environment about how to proceed. Consequently, the interruption of the motor program provides a doorway which you can utilize to create trance.

PATRICE: Is that why you speeded up verbally?

Yes, because it's also an overload induction. I'm speeding up to give a lot of instructions to overload the conscious mind, which is in a null set from the pattern interrupt. The person is then likely to go with the next suggestion—within reason—to move out of the loop. You may have noticed that initially I was actually moving his arm while I was giving the suggestion, "Look at that hand, notice the changing focus of your hand as it gets closer and closer." I was moving his hand closer to his face until it started to feel like it was getting rigid. That's the catalepsy. Then I stopped and I said, "It will get closer and you'll notice your eyes want to close," and his eyes went about halfway down. Then I gave him the nonverbal suggestion by moving my free hand downward, to close his eyes. It's a nonverbal suggestion, and it looks like you're doing something magical, but it's not magical at all once you know the structure of it.

Pattern Interrupt And Kinesthetic Ambiguity To Produce Catalepsy

Here's a similar catalepsy induction which relies on the same pattern interrupt of the automatic program and adds to it an ingredient referred to as "kinesthetic ambiguity." As you know, the use of ambiguity in language encourages TDS and the formation of trance. Kinesthetic ambiguity accomplishes the same purpose; it simply utilizes a different sensory modality. This induction is gentler, more subtle, and relies less on surprise than the previous one, and it still creates the same doorway into trance. This is our preferred method when seeing clients in our private practice. Who has a spare hand here? Dottie?

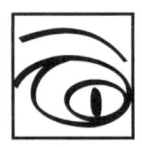

Demonstration of Pattern Interrupt And Kinesthetic Ambiguity To Produce Catalepsy

Trainer: Okay, Dottie. (To audience) Now, imagine this is being done in the context of a counseling session. I'm going to do a hypnotic induction, and what I want to do is to explain to Dottie the difference between the way the conscious mind works and the way the unconscious mind works. You already know some of these ways. One of the things which I would often explain to someone is (trainer looks at Dottie), for example, your conscious mind is functioning when you deliberately think about what you're doing or when you're paying attention to what is being said. Your unconscious handles all the things you do automatically. A lot of times, when you're in a social situation, you just do things automatically, you don't really have to think about them.

For example, if I were meeting you for the first time, and I said, "Hi, Dottie, how are you doing?" and I reach my hand up . . . . . . (Trainer lifts her hand to shake Dottie's hand. Dottie lifts her right hand and trainer gently grasps Dottie's wrist with her free, left hand.) . . . . . That arm (looking at Dottie's suspended arm) just sort of moves like that, automatically. (Spoken while trainer begins to randomly and lightly touch her wrist, sometimes giving an uncertain push upward or downward.) . . . Now, the interesting thing about that is the initial impulse is just sort of automatic. You didn't have to think consciously to make that arm move up. (Trainer applies gentle pressure upward on the word "up" while checking for development of catalepsy.) All that you had to do was just know what was expected and your arm starts to lift. Right?

... So all that I want you to do now is just notice, if you would, the tendency for that arm to start to ... just watch what I'm doing here ... so that you can notice the tendency for that hand to start to get .... (still doing random, ambiguous touch and checking for catalepsy) ..... it's starting to get almost sort of a feeling of ... right ... that's right ... it starts to get sort of that waxy kind of flexibility, a rigid kind of feeling. The thing that's really interesting ... that's right ... is that it starts to get so sort of ... if you notice these sensations in through here, they start to expand out through your hand, and it starts to get more and more stiff, and sort of wooden ... that's right ...!

... The thing that's really interesting about this wooden feeling that you don't realize yet, just as you're looking at that, is how much fun you can have learning to use that hand right there, that hand that's just nice and fixed there. I don't know what that hand would do, I don't know if the hand wants to move up or if it wants to stay where it is, or if it wants to move down for that matter. To demonstrate to you how a hypnotic arm actually works ... one of the things that you can notice, if you just watch your hand very closely, is you can begin to wonder what's going to happen first. Is that hand going to want to move up? ...... right ... that's right. .. up towards your face ... and how far is that hand going to move up? ...... Before you notice the tendency, as your eyes are fixed on that hand, for your eyes to close ... now .... you don't know which one it will be. Will your hand get to your face before your eyes close, or will your eyes close and you'll feel that hand moving up all by itself? .... (Dottie's eyes close.) .... That's right!

*Now, I would like to suggest to you, Dottie, that the hand can only begin to move up as quickly as you begin at the unconscious level ... (Trainer changes voice tone, lowers pitch, and speaks directly to Dottie's unconscious mind to create further dissociation.) ... You, her unconscious mind, can begin to consider those times in her life when she felt exquisitely **confident and competent** ... that's right ... in her own abilities ... where she might not consciously* *remember the times that you are taking her to, just yet . . . but you can perhaps find a number of times and then settle on only one that is particularly intense . . . (skin color change, breathing shift, and slight smile occurs.) . . . . . That's right . . . and notice that feeling can spread throughout all of your body . . . and in a moment, what you can begin to do is you can notice you can awaken as a mind, but not a body, so you will be able to open your eyes, and feel as though you've awakened . . . that's right . . . (Dottie opens her eyes, while her body and levitated arm remain cataleptic.)*

There's that hand there . . . it's sort of unusual to have that hand like that, isn't it? Did you ever think that you could go into a trance that way, just by looking at your hand? . . . . Now . . . . that's right . . . . very good . . . notice the tendency as that hand went down, your eyelids followed . . . that's right . . . and I don't want that hand to go down, only as quickly as that experience of utter total confidence intensifies at least fivefold . . . so that you'll know, **hands down,** *that the* **confidence is available to you whenever you want it in the future.** *We'll leave that up to your unconscious . . . that's right . . . mind to decide where and when those times can be when you'll feel bursts of extra confidence where you hadn't had it before . . . so you can have once again that experience of being surprised and delighted at yourself and your abilities . . . . (Dottie opens her eyes, reorients to her body, smiles, and nods) . . . That's right . . . !*

Pattern Interrupt And Kinesthetic Ambiguity To Produce Catalepsy Exercise

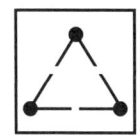

1. Begin with Conscious-Unconscious Dissociation while introducing the concept of automatic functions.

2. Then say, "For example, if we were meeting for the first time, I would walk up to you and say, 'Hi, I'm . . . . ' and offer my hand like this (extend hand to shake hands), you'd . . . . (calibrate to client lifting hand automatically) . . . . That's right!"

3. With your left hand, gently grasp the client's wrist from the outside to stabilize it.

4. Continue speaking ambiguously, while lightly touching the forearm and wrist of the client. Sometimes you can nudge it up or down with the idea of creating kinesthetic ambiguity so their conscious functions are temporarily suspended. Calibrate to the development of catalepsy.

5. Utilize to deepen trance.

Do the exercise

Discussion

The method above represents your second choice for inducing catalepsy. Essentially this particular technique begins with an explanation of conscious and unconscious processes. As you saw, if you have rapport with the client, very little Conscious-Unconscious Dissociation is needed at the beginning. Use just enough dissociation to make a smooth segue into the example of automatic processes. You can weave this in at any point in the conversation.

You could actually say, "If I was going to meet you for the first time, and I walked up to you and said, 'Hi, my name is _____,'" while extending your hand as if you're going to shake their hand.

You have to be congruent when you do this. You have to put yourself in the same state you're in when you're meeting someone and you are going to shake their hand. In a clinical setting even though you're seated, it's a good idea to change your physiology to support the quotes you're in. This is important, because you need to create the cues which will stimulate the automatic program in your client so their hand actually lifts to shake yours. Their response may vary from a slight movement to a full movement upward. It doesn't matter which response occurs as long as you get some movement. If their hand is on their lap and they lift it slightly, what do you say? "That's right." Then gently take their hand and begin doing ambiguous touch. You probably noticed I was speaking at times in incomplete sentences which were basically unintelligible; I would start an idea, and I wouldn't finish the sentence because I'm creating a maximum amount of ambiguity in a safe way. I kept doing the basic ambiguous touch until I started to feel catalepsy in her arm, a rigid kind of feeling. Once I started to observe that, then I started to suggest more of it.

Erickson did a combination of the two methods. He would do the surprise handshake induction and then he would do the ambiguous touch. Not only would he utilize surprise, he would stand there loosely grasping their hand, and doing the ambiguous touch with the fingertips of the hand with which he was shaking.

The reason we generally don't teach Erickson's method is that in this day and age, it may come across as being a bit inappropriate if you continue to hold someone's hand longer than what's usually expected—especially if you begin lightly touching their hand while you're still holding it. That may create an impression you don't want to create. That's why in our private practice we generally go with the method I used with Dottie, without using the ambiguous touch.

One final point with these types of inductions: your success in doing them will be directly proportional to *you're feeling confident that your client will go into a trance*. Both of the previous two inductions and the one we're going to do next can be rehearsed in large part without a client present. Most of the time, when people have not succeeded in doing these inductions, it's a matter of not being able to *move quickly and smoothly* after the pattern interrupt and *projecting confidence* that trance will quickly ensue.

Rehearsal Induction Using Catalepsy

This next catalepsy induction is based upon a generic rehearsal induction which has been used in hypnosis for many years. In this method, you explain to the client in a step-by-step fashion exactly what you're going to say and do and what effect it will have on them. You want to present it in a very matter-of-fact tone. You'll greatly increase the likelihood of trance when you use this format, remembering, of course, that rapport and Pacing Current Experience are presupposed.

This particular version uses rehearsal to create the same effect as the previous two catalepsy inductions. It's useful to start with this one because it doesn't require quite the same dexterity as the previous two techniques. You can literally practice it as many times as you want with your client until you decide it's time for the "real" induction. So far, although we've never gotten to the "real" induction, our clients develop catalepsy and trance! I guess we just have to keep practicing!

Demonstration of Rehearsal Induction Using Catalepsy

Trainer: Who else wants to play? Char? . . . . .

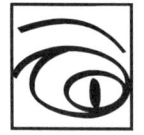

CHAR: I'd really like to, but I have difficulty going into trance and really letting go.

You'd really like to . . . that's great . . . . just stay where you are in your seat, I'll do it there. (To audience) One of the things, I don't know if Char knew this, but Erickson always used to let people know that the best hypnotic subjects were (looks directly at Char) people who sat with their hands on their lap and their feet on the floor. (Char places her hands on her lap, with her feet flat on the floor, and chuckles.) That's always worth mentioning.

All that you do is say, "Char, what I'm going to do here in a moment is I'm just going to reach over, and I'm going to pick up your hand, and I don't want you to go into trance, because I want to explain this to you . . . . . because this will be something that will assist you later in going into trance. All you're going to notice is that I'm going to pick up your wrist like this (Trainer slowly lifts her wrist) and (speaking more softly, but still quickly and conversationally) . . . . . *I'm going to talk to you in a certain way, and as that hand reaches a certain point, you'll notice a number of things happening that will let you know you're going into trance . . . . and then to have you come back out of trance, we'll move the hand back down like that* . . . (Trainer moves Char's hand back down.) *Okay?"*

(To audience) It's really pretty simple: I'm just giving her instructions. All I'm going to do—and we're not going to do it yet but I want her to get the kinesthetics—I'm just going to reach over and gently grasp her wrist and I'm going to lift it up, and at a certain point it's going to stop all by itself. Then I'm going to move it back down, okay? What we're really doing is training, or formatting, the unconscious with the exact steps for doing arm catalepsy.

So, if now's the time to do it, all I would do is to reach over like this, and (to Char) I would pick up your arm like that, and I would stop at a point when *you would go into trance, probably notice then that your eyes would close, your breathing would shift and you would go even deeper, and then have you come back out . . . that's right . . . then you would just bring this hand down like this.*

(To audience) What I'm doing now is adding a few steps. Now, if we were going to actually do it again, all I would do is reach over and I would lift that arm up like that, and when that arm stops by itself . . . *that's right* . . . (Char's arm remains suspended without assistance) . . . . *you noticed the tendency . . . not yet . . . but then you just notice the tendency for your eyes to close, and you would go deep into a trance, and once you go into a trance, all that we would do to have you come back out would be that I would push that arm back down like that.*

So that the next time when I reach over, like this (Char unconsciously anticipates trainer reaching over and begins to lift the arm herself) *That's right . . . and I would just lift up that arm . . . and it would stop all by itself . . . . .* (arm stays suspended cataleptically) *. . . . . . and you would know what to do . . . . . all the way in . . . that's right . . . that's right . . . and your unconscious mind can follow exquisitely the suggestions with your conscious mind paying attention . . .*

. . . . Now the question is how deeply into trance can you go? . . . with your eyes wide open . . . ("eyes wide open" is said increasingly more softly) *. . . How much deeper can you go with your eyes wide open? . . . That's right . . . even higher . . . I want you to stay awake . . . even more awake . . . even more awake . . . wide . . . that's right . . . wide awake . . . until it's time . . . that's right . . . now . . . all the way into a deep state . . . that's right . . . totally cataleptic . . . totally . . . notice the interruption of the eyeblink . . . the tendency for your gaze to become blurry . . . . as it becomes blurry the tendency for the eye reflex to change in some way . . .*

. . . While your conscious mind focuses on your unconscious . . . is considering times from the past . . . (Char's eyeblink has

ceased, lids are open and frozen, facial muscles have flattened)...
*When you felt **deeply secure**, felt like you were **trusting yourself**..
when you knew you were doing the right thing... by learning to
trust your unconscious, because your unconscious knows how to
dance with your conscious mind more than your conscious mind
could ever know. Your conscious mind is the part that may want to
dance, but your unconscious mind knows the steps you can take to
increase that alignment between the two just as easily. And it can
close the distance between the two so that they are one. Just as
easily as you can close the distance between that hand and your
leg.*

*Now, I only want that hand to close the distance between your
hand and your leg as quickly as the distance between your conscious and your unconscious closes and you begin to feel certain
sensations inside you can interpret as integration of being total
complete integration... peaceful... trusting... in knowing **you
can access this experience anytime you want to**.... simply by
lifting that hand on your own exactly as you did now. You can **fully
memorize this experience**, fully memorize the feelings... and
fully memorize the attitude that you can have of how closely aligned
the conscious and unconscious mind are perfectly integrated at a
level that you haven't known was possible consciously because it
needed the cooperation of your unconscious mind to do so... and
it can begin doing that now... take all the time that you need...
once that hand has closed the distance between... that's right...
you can allow your eyes to close momentarily* (Her eyes close)...
.... *Then you can*.... (Char opens her eyes and reorients.)
That's right...! You did great!

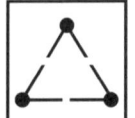

Rehearsal Induction Using Catalepsy Exercise

1. Preframe. Explain to the client that before going into a trance you want to familiarize them with the procedure you'll be using. Get permission from client before doing the technique.

2. Begin the rehearsal doing it in future quotes: "So, in a little bit, I'm going to reach over and pick up your wrist like this." (Pick up wrist at this point and begin lifting their arm.)

3. Suggest that the arm will continue to go up (as you continue to lift it) and explaining that, at some point, it will stop and the client will go into a trance.
   a. calibrate to client's physiology.
   b. intersperse any observations of your client's behavior which would support trance formation.
   c. model trance with your physiology.
   d. check if catalepsy is beginning to develop.

4. Suggest any other common behavioral manifestations of trance that could occur.

5. Begin to move the arm downward while explaining what will happen when coming out of trance.

6. Repeat Steps 1 through 5, incorporating any behavior observed in the previous rehearsal.

7. Utilize client's conditioned reflex to create catalepsy and to deepen trance.

Do the exercise

Discussion

One of the things which is useful to notice in this demonstration is how deeply a person can be in trance with their eyes wide open. At a certain point, the eyeblink reflex was totally interrupted—it just stopped—and her eyelids became cataleptic.

Catalepsy: Giving Your Trancework A Healing Lift 95

(To Char) Good job. When you have some time, I want you to go ahead and use this technique on your own, so you know you have the ability to put yourself in a trance this way whenever you want.

One of the things I noticed early on was that Char was a little bit concerned about whether she was going to be able to do it. (Char nods "yes.") I was picking up on that too. That's why I went in a slightly different direction than her normal mindset would have expected for going into trance.

This is the type of connection you want to have with your client when you do hypnosis—she knows I know what's going on, and vice versa. Her unconscious mind gives me a signal: I either get it or I don't. If I get it, I send another signal back that says, "I got that," and we just keep doing that until we get to where we want to go.

AUDIENCE: Did you do that because you were sensing resistance?

No, she was displaying behavior that we needed to match or pace. We wouldn't describe it as resistance, nor would Erickson. **We all get to experience trance in our own unique way. The only way people inadvertently stop themselves from experiencing trance is by thinking that what is happening naturally is not the right way to experience trance. Their conscious mind has expectations about how it "should" be done and that may not be the way their unconscious mind develops trance for them.**

Again, think about going into trance yourself. If you get a little nervous or excited you might think: "This better work for me." That's really okay with us because it helps motivation. It's our job as hypnotherapists to respect and utilize that so it works for the client. Actually that was a good state for Char, because she was really focusing all of her attention on what she was doing, which is the perfect trance. That's not resistance, it's resilience and persistence!

Everyone has their own way of going into trance. They'll communicate to you what that way is if you let them. Rehearsing the raising of the arm is just a starting point. How did I know when to begin the "real" trance induction? As soon as she anticipated my response: when she saw my hand coming over to pick it up, and she automatically began to lift her arm <u>before</u> I lifted it.

And I said, "That's right." What I'm doing is setting up another program just like a handshake. It's the same idea, except in this case we're teaching the program first. The program is, "I'm going to reach over and lift up your arm (as I'm picking up the arm by the wrist). You're going to notice certain things . . . your arm is going to stop there . . . . . . and then we're going to put the arm down . . . and you're going to come out of trance. Do you understand that? Let's do this a couple of times to make sure you've got it."

If she would have automatically lifted her arm the first or second time, I would have gone further into the induction. Char was so interested in being a really good subject that she was doing explicitly what I was asking her to do. Eventually we had the reflex conditioned: so when I reached over the last time, her arm went up, and I said, "That's right."

From that point on, the direction of the induction was dictated by her reaction to the suggestions which I offered her. **Utilization.** What we're calling inductions are just starting points for development of some type of response. Once you observe any of the trance behaviors, then it's up to you to pace and lead the client to move more fully into the desired state.

If you have a person who is highly intellectual, too compliant, or not comfortable experiencing trance, it's useful to know that catalepsy will often be developing in the arm to which they're paying the least attention. If you're working with the right arm the whole time, and nothing is happening with it (it may even feel like a lead weight when you lift it), this is when you say, "In a moment, that arm (right) is going to drop to your leg, and when you do, you'll feel yourself going deeper . . . ready . . . . . . now." Then let it drop as you switch to the other arm (left). You'll have displaced the mismatch by utilizing the heaviness of the arm. This generally presupposes that the other hand (left) is lighter and you can utilize that. Then you can go through the process with the arm that's left, so to speak.

As far as we're concerned, everyone knows how to do catalepsy. All of you have been doing catalepsy before you came to this seminar every day of your life. In fact, there's a part of your body that's cataleptic during probably ninety percent of your waking hours. You know what part that is? Your neck. To keep your head straight, you have to have balanced tonicity between the agonist and antagonist muscles. Everybody has the experiential understanding of catalepsy, albeit unconsciously.

CINDY: Now we're all feeling our necks . . .

And, you'll be doing that for a while . . . and that will be fine, because to the extent that you're paying attention to your neck, NOW, some other part of your body that you can't be paying attention to has just become cataleptic.

General Steps To Exercise

This is another one of those exercises where we're going to build. So, whomever you pick for this particular exercise, you'll be doing the next exercise with them. So, please pick someone with whom you haven't yet worked.

First, you will use catalepsy as an induction. Then you're going to further dissociate the conscious and unconscious minds. Once they're in a nice trance, either with their eyes open or closed, suggest to them that they can begin to wonder what other hypnotic phenomena or hypnotic skills they would like to demonstrate. Say it this way: "What other hypnotic skills would your unconscious like to develop next?" You're not necessarily expecting an answer at this point. You're asking them to consider this. To assist them, mention the ones we'll be using here: amnesia, analgesia (some people also call that glove analgesia), dissociation, and deep trance identification. Just permissively list the options: "Will it be analgesia; will it be amnesia; will it be . . . ?" and you just go down the list. They can consider which one they would like to do, because each unconscious mind may have one it would like to experience first. Pick something that's useful or fun or both.

Then, if you want, you can ask their unconscious mind to give a "yes" response once it has decided on a skill. In fact, if your partner consciously knows what their "yes" signal is, they can tell you before you induce the trance. Utilize that.

The last instruction is the final posthypnotic suggestion. You'll say, "Only come back outside once you know consciously what that hypnotic skill is, and can communicate it to me, once you awaken fully."

Catalepsy Induction And Choice of Hypnotic Phenomena Exercise

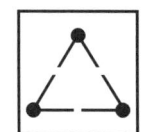

1. Induce trance and arm catalepsy.

2. Deepen trance by Pacing Current Experience and Conscious-Unconscious Dissociation.

3. Suggest: "What other hypnotic skill would your unconscious like to develop next?"
   a. go through the list of hypnotic phenomena (amnesia, dissociation, analgesia, deep trance identification).
   b. pause after each choice and calibrate to their unconscious response so you know which hypnotic skill it will be before your client tells you.

4. Ask their unconscious mind to signal with a "yes" after it has decided.

5. Posthypnotic suggestion: "Only come back outside once you know consciously what that hypnotic skill is, and can communicate it to me, once you awaken fully."

Do the exercise

Discussion

Welcome back. How many of you noticed that this trance can be kind of an uplifting experience that can be handy for you?

Let me suggest a couple of things as refinements. A faster way is ..... (trainer looks at co-trainer) ...... can I borrow your arm? It's far more effective if you <u>move your touch</u> around on the forearm and wrist when you're inducing catalepsy. This technique creates the same effect kinesthetically that the Milton Model does with language. Continuing to vary your touch will temporarily suspend the conscious mind because it won't know what is going to happen next and that's what you want to accomplish. If you keep your hand in the same place the whole time, your client is getting a clear communication from you. Their conscious mind can be directly involved in that. However, if first you very subtly push it up, then move it to the side, then move it to the other side, or touch the fingers, moving them up and moving them down, and then finally going back over to the forearm, you'll produce ambiguity. All the while, they're consciously thinking, "Is the arm supposed to go up or go down or what? What is it supposed to be doing?"

DON: I got catalepsy up to my elbow, but my shoulder felt very heavy, I could feel up in here that it wasn't particularly comfortable, but my lower arm was fine. The other thing was I wasn't sitting in a chair when I was the subject.

If you want, you can suggest that the client's arm can position itself in a way that can be totally comfortable and that the comfort can spread throughout his/her entire arm, the whole way up into the shoulder, the neck, and throughout the entire body.

This is a worthwhile experience for you to have in training because otherwise you might not know that clients may have experiences like that. If you're in a chair, and your elbow is already positioned on the armrest, it's much easier—your shoulder generally won't feel anything because your shoulder is already resting as your body's resting.

Traditional hypnotists might suggest something like, "Imagine that there's a shelf on which your arm's comfortably resting." You can use presupposition to strengthen that suggestion. "What kind of shelf is that? Is that a metal shelf, is it wood, maybe hardwood, or pine? Just imagine that your arm is resting on that shelf, in fact your whole body, even your shoulder can just lean on that and very comfortably rest on that shelf—it's nice to have things to support you; we all need that."

SAM: I really noticed as my one arm was going up, my other arm was feeling heavier and heavier.

This is something that the traditional hypnotists knew and it does happen fairly frequently—we usually perceive one arm as being heavier than the other. It's actually a leverage point, when you're doing catalepsy or arm levitation, because you can say to the person, "I want you to notice the difference between the lightness in one arm compared to the other." When they notice it, their conscious mind notes, "Oh, gosh, he's right." That's another thing which you can utilize.

Remember trance is an amplifier, so generally, what was already present is going to be amplified. That contrast in arm weight also becomes amplified. One of the easiest ways to handle the situation when one arm is not going up is to say, "That's right . . . it's not going up . . . it's getting heavier . . . it's getting so heavy that it's considerably heavier than the hand that's left . . . and who knows which one is the right one for you because your right could be my left, and I don't know which one would be the left one that will really be the right one to lift up NOW."

You can take whichever hand is experiencing the heaviness and go with that and put all the person's attention on that hand. Then move right on to lifting the other one because it will probably be cataleptic.

In our introductory course in hypnosis, we teach the "brick and balloon" suggestibility test. We ask people to extend their arms out in front of them with the right hand turned palm up. We tell them to imagine holding a heavy brick in that hand. Next, we instruct them to make a fist with their left hand and point their thumb up toward the ceiling. Tied to the thumb is a string attached to several helium balloons. So as that hand is being lifted by the balloons, the hand holding the brick is becoming heavier and heavier.

This test is based on a predictable physiological reflex that results from the specific positioning of the hands. If your arms are extended and you place one palm up, there will be a natural tendency for that arm to want to lower. Making a fist with the thumb tensed and pointing upward creates the tendency for that arm to lift, especially if suggestions are timed to the subject's inhalations.

Once the hands start to separate and you've got some type of movement, you can suggest that the heavier the right arm becomes, the lighter the left arm will become. The contrast effect working here tends to exaggerate the relative heaviness of the right hand and the relative lightness of the left hand. Erickson called this "apposition of opposites."[8]

Regardless of how easily you *produce catalepsy,* you have a versatile hypnotic skill that has a wide range of application. We use it for smoking cessation, weight loss, self-hypnosis, and a number of other issues. For example, it's easy to use if you have a headache and want to let go of it naturally. You just put yourself in trance, give yourself the suggestion that your unconscious mind will come up with all the alternatives for getting rid of your headache . . . *as your arm lifts*. Ask it to have your arm lower only at the rate that it implements the alternatives and clears your head. Give yourself about fifteen minutes to do this. Regarding smoking and weight loss, we use catalepsy and self-hypnosis as ways to have resources available if urges occur. These are just a few ideas which can stimulate other ideas.

COLETA:
>Would the catalepsy be useful with somebody who's struggling with a lot of back and neck pain?

It can be. When people come in and they have pain, their pain is a form of trance. If you begin to induce relaxation or dissociation before they can adequately separate from the pain, they'll report that they can't go into trance. It's because moving from pain to relaxation may be too large of a leap. You have to use the pain as the point of fixation as you begin the trance induction. It is occupying their attention, so you might as well use it. Erickson discusses this extensively in *Healing in Hypnosis*.[9]

What you're learning now in regard to pain is a set of generic skills which you can embellish with your own creativity. I'll share with you a personal example of working with acute dental pain. I went through the procedure where they remove all of the silver amalgams from your teeth. I had thirty-six separate fillings drilled out and replaced over the course of six visits. I did the whole process without any novocaine and I only had nitrous oxide on two occasions, for less than a total of ten minutes. I used self-hypnosis and catalepsy to create dissociation. Catalepsy can be used to easily facilitate partial or total dissociation. When the dentist drilled, I could hear the drill and I could tell where he was working. I could feel sensation and it wasn't pain. I just used simple *dissociation* which, by the way, is one of the hypnotic skills we'll be discussing and *developing more fully for you* during the next section. Today when I talk about it, I still feel very empowered by the experience because it is something which I did all on my own. It was a great convincer for my conscious mind of the value of trance and unconscious rapport, and since it was a dental issue that was a real test.

Catalepsy and Healing

At the beginning of this chapter, we mentioned that catalepsy may also have applications for physiological healing. We believe there is a plausible if not actual connection between mechanisms involved in catalepsy and physiological healing. Before we discuss this, we ought to mention that we as therapists don't heal clients. People heal themselves. After being cleared medically and or diagnosed by a physician, we can help the client remove the symptoms which were associated with the underlying dis-ease [sic] process. We can also help them clear any impediments which may have prevented them from healing in a natural and timely manner. However, the client does the healing.

Oftentimes we'll use catalepsy metaphorically as the basis of healing. Most people consider healing to be an automatic process—something over which they don't have voluntary control. By assisting a person in experiencing catalepsy, analgesia, and anesthesia (lack of pain or lack of sensation, respectively), you assist them in expanding what is possible for self-healing. Most people in our culture equate healing with the lack of pain. That's not necessarily an accurate understanding, although it is a widely accepted notion within the lay public. Many people believe that when pain goes away, *healing is occurring*. Removing or reducing pain opens a doorway for more pervasive, generative changes in the healing process.

In hypnosis, it's not what's logical that matters, it's whether it's plausible. Plausibility is what works at the unconscious level.[10] It seems plausible to most people that if they have voluntary control over something which was previously an involuntary response, they will be able to control other so-called "involuntary" functions in their body. Mainstream thought suggests that you can assist healing, but the actual, internal process of healing itself is beyond conscious control. Our role is to provide counterexamples to this type of thinking. The most compelling counterexamples are experiential—those which are amenable to the senses. Catalepsy and analgesia, when used this way, can create compelling experiences which then form the foundation for new beliefs about one's ability to heal.

Sometimes I'll state this directly to the person. *"You didn't think before we did this that you would be capable of having analgesia in your arm, but* **now** *you know* **you can produce these kinds of healing effects** *in your body. I don't know what other parts of your body would be in need of this same kind of healing. I don't know what other functions of your body you can learn to use purposely. Perhaps you haven't fully realized that at the cellular level, each and every cell of your body can live as a single-cell organism. Each cell has its own intelligence. And each cell is directly in communication with your unconscious mind via neuropeptides. So, it will be interesting to discover just* *when **your unconscious** will begin transferring these abilities from this arm to another part of your body in such a way that the other part of your body can respond in the same way and **can heal.**"*

That's what we usually tell our clients who want to heal something, but we probably don't need to tell <u>you</u> that **now**, because you already understand how to give your trancework a healing **lift**. **Cataleptically.**

Chapter 6
Hypnotically Skillfull

Editor's Notes: This section occurs at the halfway point in the training. The momentum continues to build as the trainers preframe hypnotic phenomena as "skills." Some students of Hypnosis seem to find these skills intimidating and thus never learn them. One of the "meta" outcomes for this section is to normalize these skills, so that the participants view them as naturally occurring experiences and pathways for communication with their unconscious minds.

The reader may want to note the "holographic" nature of the Deep Trance Identification (DTI) induction, where the sequence of embedded suggestions alone represents the totality of this pattern. The reader may notice that the embedded suggestions continue after the formal DTI induction is complete. There is one primary exercise in which the client chooses a particular hypnotic phenomenon to experience. The development of the "skill" occurs via association which is one Ericksonian approach to elicit classical phenomena. Both direct and indirect suggestions are used to accomplish the elicitation.

This chapter, therefore, represents one of the primary objectives of this work: to blend Ericksonian techniques with traditional hypnotic phenomena so the hypnotherapist has many choices for assisting clients to change.

We remember wondering, during our early days in Hypnosis training, when would we finally get to the "heavy stuff," the hypnotic phenomena? Such things as amnesia, analgesia, hallucination, and age regression. (Those were the only ones we knew about at the time!) Learning these techniques seemed really exciting—could we actually induce a positive hallucination? Think of all the things we could use amnesia for... I forget what they are now, but they seemed important at the time! Beyond the "novelty" of these techniques lies their true value: they are pointers to the vast, deep, and often untapped potential we all have. They literally act as "convincers" for our conscious mind to recognize that we have far greater abilities than we think we do. They assist us in recognizing capabilities which reach beyond our ordinary, everyday mindsets. Mastering hypnotic phenomena, both as a clinician and as an hypnotic subject, increases the likelihood that we will utilize our unconscious mind in a more purposeful way. When we tap this hidden potential, it may also assist us in establishing a more self-reliant and generative approach to life.

In therapy, the elicitation of hypnotic phenomena, and the clients' recognition of them, can be a graphic metaphor of the ability to uncover the resources of the unconscious mind. *Like trance* itself, these skills occur naturally in daily life; we simply overlook them. Because of this, few people appreciate what an extraordinary set of generic skills they are, and consequently, few people *fully develop* them as part of their behavioral repertoire.

As we discuss these hypnotic skills, it's interesting to note that many newcomers to Hypnosis are concerned about losing control during hypnosis. This is a common misconception and is far from the truth. What is commonly understood and experienced by those who utilize these skills is that they *gain control* from using them—control over parts of their bodies and nervous systems which people ordinarily think are not within their conscious control.

Gaining control can be a very effective reframe to use with clients. You might ask them, "Wouldn't you want the ability to deal with pain in a different way from using chemicals? Wouldn't it be useful to do that, or to intensify positive feelings when you want to, and to separate yourself from feelings which aren't comfortable?" Explaining to them that these hypnotic skills can be utilized to gain control of such things as headaches, constant muscular discomfort, and sports injuries, as well as preparation for and healing after a surgical procedure, is often a convincer. The possibilities for application are endless. They underscore your ability to take charge of your "bodymind" and improve its functioning through your own powers.

One of the more useful exercises which will greatly enhance your hypnotic abilities is to identify everyday examples of these skills. To the extent you have examples of hypnotic phenomena which are universal experiences, you can use those universals to activate associations in your client before you make any direct suggestion to elicit the actual phenomenon. Here's a brief overview providing a definition of the hypnotic phenomena and corresponding universals. We have also included trance and catalepsy, which have been covered previously, in order to complete the list.

Overview of Classic Hypnotic Phenomena

• Trance

What would be an everyday example of trance occuring naturally in our lives? When we're driving: specifically when we're taking a long drive on the freeway. How about when you pull up to a red light and you're waiting for the light to change—and you don't notice the light has changed until you hear the driver behind you honk his horn? That's an example. Elevators may also be excellent trance inducers. Being in a supermarket can induce a definite trance state—while you're waiting in the checkout line with nothing to do other than wait (in trance)!

It's useful to have a collection of these examples. Once you've chosen some, you can expand on them when you're working with your clients. The more universal or common the examples are, the better they work. For example, almost everyone drives a car these days and has waited at a red light. Most everyone has been to the supermarket or waited in a line somewhere. Most everyone has watched TV—that's a favorite American trance!

• Catalepsy

Catalepsy is a condition where balanced tonicity exists between the agonist and antagonist muscles—arm levitation is an example. In hypnosis, when catalepsy occurs and arm levitation is suggested, it feels as if your arm is lifting itself involuntarily. That's because your unconscious mind is lifting it for you. Therefore the kinesthetics and the proprioceptive senses are quite different from what you experience when you lift your arm voluntarily.

As my arm moves up (trainer demonstrates with arm while in an autohypnotic trance), notice that it moves relatively slowly, in small jerky movements, almost as if it's being lifted by a winch. If you look at my fingers now, they're somewhat extended and pretty firm as my whole hand is becoming cataleptic. If at this point you provided a suggestion for my arm to stay suspended right where it is, and you try to push it up or down, it would simply stay where it is.

What are some naturally occurring events where you would see someone experiencing arm catalepsy? Holding a cigarette. If you wanted a healthier example where else might you experience this? How about eating? Think of someone engaged in conversation and as they lift their fork they stop in midair to finish what they're saying. They're ready to take that bite and they hold it there so long that you're ready to eat it for them! That's catalepsy. While they're deeply engaged in the conversation, they're not aware of their arm. For that moment, their arm is dissociated from the other feelings in their body. If we caught them right at that moment and asked them about their arm they might have a funny feeling like, "Is that really my arm suspended there?"

In fact, we could use this as an example of both dissociation and catalepsy. Catalepsy is simply when a body part manifests waxy flexibility. Waxy flexibility is an old psychiatric term for catatonia. The dissociation aspect begins to emerge as a result of conscious awareness being distracted from a particular body part. Subsequently, when conscious attention is refocused on that part and appropriate suggestions are made, the client will have the experience of being detached from that body part, or even in some cases, their entire body.

The fourth hypnotic skill is time distortion.

We didn't do number three. Did you do amnesia?

I wanted to give you an example!

• Time distortion

We're looking for two classes of examples: 1) experiences when things went very fast for someone and time went by very quickly and 2) experiences when things went very slowly and time just seemed to crawl. What are some universal experiences of these two categories? Watching a great movie, taking a day off from work, or doing anything that you really enjoyed and wanting it to last longer are all examples of time seeming to speed up. Counterexamples would be anytime you've been bored or impatient: listening to a speaker drone on, going on a long drive, or waiting for that special someone to arrive and it seems like forever.

Here's something to consider if you're wondering where time distortion would be useful. Consider how much fun it would be to take a great experience where the time seemed to go by too fast and then associate to that experience the resource of time moving ever so slowly so you can enjoy the great experience even longer! You can take each of the two experiences above (fast time/slow time) and switch the submodalities[1] so the great experiences slow down and the not-so-great experiences speed by in no time.

Time distortion is also very effective for pain relief. For most people in pain, time drags on because they are so aware of the pain. If you found out how to speed things up for them, they could have eight hours of pain in one minute. This was a technique which Erickson used extensively. He would set it up so they would have excruciating pain for one minute, and since he wouldn't take away the pain completely, that would handle the issue of ecology. In this case you don't have to actually find out what the highest intention of the pain is because you're not eliminating the pain. In most cases the secondary gain, generally speaking, remains intact.

Alternatively, what if you hypnotically refresh an experience where time just dragged on and associate the submodalities of slowness to a time when time went much too fast? We'll let you think of what "stimulating moments" could be pleasantly lengthened!

It's worth watching one of Erickson's most famous videotapes, *The Monde Tape*, because he does that with her. He has her experience a number of spankings which occurred in her childhood in the time it takes her to close and reopen her eyes. By the time she opens her eyes, the process of reliving it is complete.[2]

• Analgesia and anesthesia

Analgesia is the absence of pain and the ability to still sense pressure if applied. Anesthesia is the total lack of sensation, including the inability to sense pressure. We teach both of these phenomena, and we tend to use analgesia more frequently for pain control in therapy. Analgesia is much easier to accomplish, because the sensation of pressure remains. If I reached over and touched Lee and she had analgesia, she could feel the pressure of my touch against her skin but she would not feel the sensation of pain. Anesthesia is total numbness: no feeling whatsoever. Experiences of analgesia and anesthesia occur when we use certain medications such as aspirin and novocaine, or when we're out in the freezing cold and our hands become numb, or when we sit in a certain position and a part of our body "falls asleep."

• Dissociation

Dot modeled this very nicely for everyone. Dissociation is where you have the sense of being detached from a part or from all of your body. In one of the earlier audience demonstrations, Dot said, "I don't feel my body." If she's not feeling her body, she must be dissociated from her body. Dissociation happens commonly in dreams, where you find yourself seeing yourself in the dream, as you're existing only as a mind. Universal examples of dissociation would be any time you see your reflection in a window or a mirror, watching yourself on videotape, or dreaming. In dreams, we often experience ourselves as consciousness without the experience of our bodies.

• Disorientation of time

Disorientation of time is literally when you don't know what time it is. Consider situations where you temporarily weren't sure what time it was, where your judgment of time was temporarily suspended or impaired. Have you ever awakened from a nap and weren't sure what time it was? Have you ever awakened in the morning and not known if it was a work day or a day off? The experience of déjà vu is also an example of disorientation of time.

• Disorientation of space

This is an impairment or suspension of judgment relative to location or space. Again, have you ever awakened in the morning or from a nap (this can happen easily if you travel a lot) and asked yourself, "Where am I today?" Or have you ever been on a long drive and for a moment lost track of exactly where you were? These are both examples of spatial disorientation.

• Disorientation of body

This is when your proprioception, or your body sense, is temporarily suspended or greatly diminished. Proprioception is your ability to know and to coordinate where different parts of your body are in relation to the rest of your body, and knowing what one part of your body is doing in relation to the other. This can often occur in trance as a concomitant of catalepsy. An example is learning a new physical skill, such as playing the piano. How do you keep track of what each finger of each hand is doing? Infants contend with bodily disorientation until they reach a developmental age where they form a map of their bodies. How about walking up steps and thinking there's another step and it's not there? That would be another example of body disorientation.

• Positive hallucination

A positive hallucination is not just a hallucination that you like! A positive hallucination is seeing, hearing, feeling, smelling, or tasting something which everyone else would agree isn't there. Interestingly, when most everyone else agrees that it's there, it's not a hallucination anymore. This is the basis of the mental health system in America—when enough people hallucinate the same thing, then it's true!

Some of you have been deep enough in trance that you've added steps to the instructions which we gave you and you carried out those hallucinated steps in the exercise. That's an example of a positive auditory hallucination. One of the easiest ways to pace and lead positive visual hallucination is to utilize the effect of afterimages and build on them. Staring at a candle and looking away is an experience which will activate associations that will support the formation of positive visual hallucinations. Tastes and smells may be induced by utilizing conditioned responses and simply mentioning the stimulus, like the smell of chocolate chip cookies baking in the oven.

• Negative hallucination

This occurs when you don't see, hear, feel, smell, or taste something everybody else would agree is there. What's the most common day-to-day example we all refer to? Have you ever had important papers which just decided to hide from you? Sometimes even while you were looking right at them! Keys are another common one. We were doing a seminar in Hawaii once and I was pretty tranced out. I had to go up to our hotel room and I had my hands full. I went all the way to our room on the seventh floor and realized I didn't have my keys. I thought to myself, "Where are the keys?" I put down all the stuff I was carrying and looked through this pouch I have. Finally, I moved my head down far enough and realized I was holding the keys in my mouth! That was a deep trance!

A distinction which we'd like to make here, which is something that's not often considered, is that for every positive hallucination there is a negative hallucination. For you to positively hallucinate an apple in my hand, you would have to negatively hallucinate the part of my hand which would be obscured by the apple. And for every negative hallucination, there has to be a positive hallucination. They always occur in pairs.

• Deep trance identification

This is one of our favorite ones. Deep Trance Identification (DTI) is the process whereby you literally assume psychologically, in part or in whole, the identity of someone else. This is particularly useful when you find someone who is an exquisite model of something which you want to incorporate into your own behavior. You begin DTI by first learning everything you possibly can about the person whom you're modeling. You read everything about them and watch videos if possible. Then you have someone assist you into trance and float over into the person whom you're modeling, taking with you all of your data about them so you have that as a point of reference. Then you begin to experience the world as that person does. For the sake of ecology, you float out of that person and bring back all of your learnings as you reintegrate into your own body. Then you begin doing the new behaviors you've just modeled.

What's an example of DTI which people do all the time? Kids look up to their Dad and think, "My Dad's my hero; I love my Dad; he's the best dad." They DTI with Dad. On occasion if a young girl does that with Dad, and Dad slips up and she realizes he's not perfect, she may react by saying he's destroyed her faith in men. If she DTI'd strongly with him and put him on a pedestal, and then she discovers he's human, it may not be easy for either one of them.

To some extent the process of NLP modeling is the denominalization of Deep Trance Identification. The New Behavior Generator,[3] one of the early NLP patterns, produces a DTI-like experience. DTI is one of the primary phenomena occurring when we watch movies and read novels. We begin to feel the emotions of the actors—we "identify" with them. Method acting is based upon the principle of Deep Trance Identification.

• Age regression

Age regression is the reaccessing and complete revivification of past memories or the complete accessing and return to an earlier period of development. Spontaneous age regression is one of the main reasons clients come to therapy. Spontaneous age regression occurs when we respond to someone in our present life in the same or similar manner in which we responded to parents, teachers, or authority figures when we were much younger. Classroom learning situations often create spontaneous age regressions, particularly if the person has negative anchors associated to the learning context. Talking "baby talk" will also spontaneously regress some people.

The information in the above categories is intended to prime the pump and assist you in finding your own examples of hypnotic skills, or what are classically referred to as hypnotic phenomena. We're going to focus on four of these skills during this training in trance: amnesia, dissociation, analgesia, and Deep Trance Identification. We could give you other common examples of these skills, but that would defeat our purpose. Once you have examples from your personal history, you'll be much more congruent and effective when you want to elicit them from others. In fact, just having a conviction that everyone experiences these skills, backed up with your own reference experience of them, will often compensate for any lack of technical skill you may have. The work of George Estabrooks, a contemporary of Erickson, suggested that the client will not actualize what the therapist does not believe.[4] Stating this in the positive, **your clients will actualize what you yourself believe.** One of our beliefs, which we want you all to realize, is *you're great hypnotic subjects.* Our experience is that the **best hypnotic subjects make the best hypnotherapists.** We know you all want to be great hypnotherapists or you wouldn't have bothered to *continue learning* all that you have up to this point. Just continue to ***trans-fer*** your *learnings* and they'll be there when you need them.

Later on, you're going to do an induction and elicit catalepsy. Catalepsy is useful to elicit because it gives you a gauge for the level of trance which your clients are experiencing. It is also an analog ideomotor signal which you can use to monitor the rate at which they complete a particular task while in trance. For example, you can ask their unconscious mind to raise the arm only as quickly as it can *find those times of exquisite confidence.* This gives you a way to measure where they are in the task, rather than just having digital "yes" and "no" signals.

In the case of dissociation, catalepsy is directly useful because when people experience catalepsy, they may also feel dissociated from their arm, like "it's somebody else's arm out there." In the case of analgesia, catalepsy is vital. It's the easiest way to produce analgesia or anesthesia. Analgesia can be a natural by-product of arm catalepsy.

After inducing trance and catalepsy, you'll assist your partner in accessing whichever hypnotic skill they decided they wanted to develop from the last exercise. We're going to discuss a structure which is particularly effective for eliciting hypnotic phenomena. First, you'll **activate associations through examples.** This is why we asked you earlier to find examples of these from your personal history that are universal experiences. You want to have two or three everyday examples of the particular phenomenon which you can utilize while your partner's in trance. Then you'll **pace and lead** your partner toward the desired response. You'll be using their current experience to assist them in developing the hypnotic phenomenon. Finally, after you have some verification that the phenomenon which they have selected is beginning to occur, **directly suggest** its occurrence.

Elicitation of Hypnotic Phenomena And Posthypnotic Suggestion

a. **Provide universal examples** to activate the appropriate neural networks.

b. **Pace and lead** the client's current experience toward the desired response. (This serves as the bridge between the associations activated in a. and the direct suggestions in c.)

c. **Directly suggest** the desired response only after you have sensory verification of its development. (Remember as you're proceeding in this process the likelihood is that steps a. and b. above are going to deepen the trance. The deeper you go, the more direct you want to become. Once you've elicited the response, use direct suggestion thereafter. It will save you a lot of time!)

Examples To Set Up Analgesia

Let's say you want to elicit analgesia. A common example is the numbing effect of novocaine. For anybody who wants to experience analgesia in this group, is there anyone who didn't have novocaine or experience some other local anesthetic? Everybody has experienced it? Okay, that's pretty universal for this group anyway. Another one is—did you ever have the experience where you took a nap or were just lying down for awhile and your arm fell asleep? Have you ever applied ice to a part of your body and noticed what happens? Another related class of examples comes from the nervous system's predilection toward desensitization and habituation with any constant stimulus. An example of this is wearing watches; most people are no longer aware of them because they have habituated to the sensation of the watch on their arm.

Here's one you can do right now. Take some loose skin on your forearm and squeeze it hard enough to feel a little discomfort. Tug at it a bit. Now touch that part of your forearm with your finger and you'll notice that the sensitivity decreases quite a bit. (Repeat as necessary.) You can do something like this as a reference experience for your client before you begin the actual induction.

One of the things we know about the nervous system is that it is designed to detect change in our environment. When something remains constant over a period of time, we begin to delete that information.[5] This can also be the basis for creating negative hallucinations. Have you ever been in a situation where there was a fan on, and at first you were aware of the fan, and then you became absorbed with something and you realized later that while you were absorbed you no longer heard the fan? Let's say that you hang a new picture on the wall, and for awhile you notice it every time you enter the room. However, as time goes on your attention is drawn to other things in the room. You've become desensitized, and you've habituated to that stimulus. Your brain says, "There's nothing new that's happening here, so we don't have to pay attention to that anymore." That's another way of producing an analgesic effect through a negative hallucination. Oops, but we told you we weren't going to have you actually do negative hallucinations here!

Another final class of examples used to elicit analgesia is based upon distraction. This happens all the time with headaches. Have you ever had a headache and went to see action-packed thriller or watched an exciting game on TV, or become really engaged in a deep conversation? Then, at some point later you discovered your headache was gone or greatly reduced? Those are fairly universal examples. Here's one that's not universal, but it works the same way. One of Dr. Erickson's more famous pain relief cases involved a woman who was bedridden with pain. He looked at her and said, "Madam, if

I told you that a lean, hungry tiger was lurking beneath your bed, what would happen to your pain?" She says, "It would be gone . . . (and then realizes to her surprise) . . . . it is gone!"[6] Now that's distraction!

Now you'll notice that distraction may not be directly related to feeling numbness in a part of your body, but examples like this support it, and that's what you're looking for. You may discover that sometimes it's easier to combine several hypnotic phenomena to get your end result. For example, a fair percentage of folks will **experience analgesia spontaneously** while experiencing catalepsy. You can utilize this knowledge. To stack the deck, first describe some common examples of analgesia while you're getting catalepsy. You can easily combine these two skills as you're doing the induction. Once you have some recognition on their part that they have had experiences like you're describing, then suggest that their arm will move up or down only as quickly as they begin to consider other similar times which they've experienced. After they have completed that, have them open their eyes while remaining in trance and begin to question them about what they're noticing in their arm. **Pace and lead** them to analgesia. You could say, ". . . And what are you noticing about your arm?" They say, "Nothing." You say, "That's right, you're feeling nothing (**pace**) . . . . in the same way after the novocaine has begun to work . . . Now . . . You understand that, don't you?" (**lead**)

Let's pretend they say, "I feel a tingly feeling in my fingers." You say, ". . . A tingly feeling in your fingers (pace) . . . . and how much are you noticing that tingly feeling is spreading to your wrist or your arm?" (lead) If they notice it, you say, "That's right (pace) and that tingly feeling can remind you of other sensations (lead) . . . . and what did it feel like when the novocaine starts to spread?"

If they say they don't notice the tingly feeling spreading, that's fine, just say, "That's right, you don't notice it's spreading, you don't notice it at all (pace) . . . . How many other times have you not noticed sensations in one part of your body? (lead) It's easy to do when you're interested in thinking about . . . . . (some pleasant distraction) . . . . "

Get how this works? The possibilities are endless. However they respond is perfect because it's a message to you about how they're going to access the phenomenon (analgesia in this case). It makes it much easier if you have already given examples of analgesia before you question them about their experience. You've already lit up the neural networks which you're going to lead them to as part of the questioning process. Then you take them through the experience, using their current sensory experience as the vehicle. Once you have some acknowledgment on their part that they're experiencing the phenomenon, **then** you **suggest its occurrence directly.** This is an extremely effective way to combine the best of indirect and direct suggestions and increase the odds of their efficacy.

Ecology And Analgesia

There are several points to consider when you're using analgesia to reduce or eliminate pain. Unless you're a physician, it is important to make sure your client has been cleared medically before you do this in a clinical setting. Pain is a signal and its message needs to be checked out before doing anything to take it away.

Even if a client has been cleared by their physician, it is appropriate to secure an agreement with their unconscious mind that it will recreate the pain whenever the client either tries to engage in counterproductive physical activity, or if there is some other reason that he or she should seek medical attention. I've done a fair amount of work in assisting injured athletes to accelerate their healing after surgery. In most cases, pain control was something which they wanted. Sometimes, the very reason why they injured themselves was because they ignored their own pain signals. Therefore, it was usually necessary to work with them first on resolving those issues. Other times it was important to get their unconscious cooperation in following through with the rehabilitation regimen they were given. In most cases, the important thing was restoring their level of confidence and what some refer to as "body confidence," which is just another way of saying "trusting your unconscious mind." Trance is certainly useful for that!

A final point has to do with the psychological aspect of pain. Only take away the pain that is acceptable to take away. You can ask the unconscious mind to do that, by the way. The mistake that some hypnotherapists make when first attempting pain reduction work is that they try to take all the pain away. First of all, you want to investigate what part it plays in their inner and outer life. In NLP, we would talk about discovering the highest intention of the pain. In the case of chronic pain, it is not unusual to find secondary gain. If you suggest total abolition of the pain, most of the time it is temporary, if there is any relief at all. You can read about what Erickson did in the *Collected Papers of Milton H. Erickson M.D.* He usually would change the nature of the pain.[7] He might move the pain around or have the person experience one minute of excruciating pain each morning when they wake up by using time distortion, rather than having them feel the pain all day. That way, it tended to keep the ecology intact because any psychological benefits from the pain would be preserved. The pain would be in a form which would seem more tolerable.

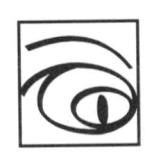

Elicitation of Dissociation

Trainer: Just for fun, here's a brief technique using dissociation. Does anybody have a mild headache?

DON: I've got chronic tension in my forehead. I get it when I project (worry) about doing this (the next exercise).

Trainer: Great, so you can get in touch with it right now? (Trainer waits for Don's acknowledgment.) . . . . So what I want you to do is . . . . . . to go ahead and see a mirror . . . Now . . . See yourself in the mirror . . . . Okay? (Trainer waits for Don's acknowledgment.) Where's the pain now?

(Don looks perplexed and says nothing.)

Trainer: Now check.

DON: It's not there.

Trainer: Are you sure? Double-check. (To audience) He's having trouble finding it. (To Don) Well, *you projected this time and it **disappeared**.* Dissociation. When you see yourself in a mirror, you're dissociated. That's the pattern. It's got to be something very situational like this. Make sure you've got rapport before you do it to increase the acceptance of the suggestions. Just ask them to see themselves in the mirror, and then ask very quickly, as soon as they access that, ask, "Where is the pain now?"

Another time when the dissociation mirror metaphor is useful is in removing an unwanted feeling temporarily or completely. Again, when using dissociation to clear a state, make sure to handle the ecology. It's a good idea to ask the person what they need to learn from the feeling. The mirror is a great universal example because you have the interesting advantage of having the person associated looking at themselves dissociated. It gives you a lot of flexibility to go either way depending on what's needed.

What is referred to as V-K (Visual-Kinesthetic) Dissociation[8] in the NLP community has roots in Erickson's work[9,10] as well as that of some of his contemporaries.[11] He used the theater metaphor—sitting in the audience and watching a memory like a movie on the screen. The idea is to separate the visual and (usually by presupposition) the auditory component of the memory from the kinesthetics. If you need additional dissociation, suggest that their body can remain comfortably seated while they float up, as an objective mind, into the projection booth and watch the movie from there. As many of you know, this has been one of the most effective techniques in NLP and is known as the phobia or trauma model. It's something that every therapist ought to have in her or his toolbox. (If you want a more detailed account, see the Appendix.)

The most important point about dissociation is that people need to learn something from the point of view of being an objective, dissociated mind with all of the resources they currently have. That's right out of Time Line Therapy ™.[12] Does anybody else have any other examples of dissociation?

DOT: Isn't denial a form of dissociation?

Yes, it can be a form of dissociation. However, the root of it is massive association, usually to some form of trauma or memories which are unpleasant. What you're talking about is repression. I wouldn't use this as an example, because what is underneath the dissociation and the repression of the memory is association to severe trauma. A person may dissociate from the memory because they're storing the memory just like they are there, like it's happening (associated). Their unconscious mind has to completely repress it to insulate them from the traumatic feelings.

This brings up a good point. You want to consider what context you are using when you're presenting the examples of dissociation to your client. Depending on the context, like everything else, we can judge it as being positive or not, i.e., is it currently beneficial to the individual?

People who are heavily associated to physical or emotional pain have difficulty functioning. Interrupting the pain to gain distance and perspective makes them resourceful. For my dental work, I needed a bit more distance to be resourceful. Dissociation which is based upon repression, where you have a dissociated personality (with parts or fragments) occurring because the person has been traumatized, is different from dissociation as we are utilizing it in this case.

Boredom will often produce dissociation. The mind wants stimulation. It says, "I'm not getting anything here," so it goes somewhere else. An obvious way to create dissociation is through Conscious-Unconscious Dissociation. Another way is with Revivification. If you have a person reliving an experience which they were in before, they aren't here. If they are associated to a pleasant memory somewhere else, they're dissociated from here. Daydreaming and night dreaming are other examples of dissociation. Night dreaming is a great one for amnesia, too. Dreams in general are a great presuppositional kind of suggestion for a number of hypnotic phenomena.

Have you ever looked at a picture of yourself and thought, "That doesn't really look like me or look the way I picture myself." That's dissociation. Hearing yourself on tape often produces the same response. Another example is when someone says to you, "You said such-and-such," and you say, "I didn't say that, did I? That doesn't sound like something I would say." Dissociation occurs where there's distance between whatever you think you are as the subject and the object which is portrayed outside of you.

Dissociation opens the door for other hypnotic skills.[13] Take Deep Trance Identification (DTI) for instance. The basis of DTI is association, so dissociation is a good setup for DTI. Another easy way to elicit analgesia via dissociation is to suggest *as you're processing what I'm communicating, now, you can wake up and be alert from the neck up while noticing that your body can remain comfortably immobile and asleep. You can feel as though you can awaken as a mind but not a body.* This will often produce or maintain catalepsy, analgesia, and/or anesthesia.

There are a number of nuances in your delivery which will greatly enhance any dissociation which you're suggesting. The primary tools you have to create and stabilize dissociation are spatial and temporal prepositions, verb tenses, pronouns, and your voice locus, to name a few. Let's say you want to have your client see themselves on a movie screen.

Starting with just spatial prepositions and voice locus, I might say, "As you're sitting here with me I'm sure there have been times when you've been in a movie theater. You know what that's like . . . " (while projecting my voice locus toward the client sitting with me, voice locus 1) . . . "I wonder if you could see a blank movie screen over there (projecting voice locus out in front of client, voice locus 2). (1) " . . . . And can you notice just how comfortable you can continue being, sitting in this chair, (2) while you can look out at that screen over there?"

Now I can add in tenses and say, (1) "I don't know how clearly you can see . . . (2) that younger you on that screen who experienced that memory, (1) . . . but I do know you're an adult now and (2) that was a long time ago."

Now adding the pronoun distinctions to the tenses and temporal prepositions and voice locus, I might say, (1) " . . . And it's comforting to notice how much more you know now . . . (2) than she knew then . . . . . . "

If you wanted to create double dissociation, you would add a third voice locus and a higher pitch for the projection booth that would be above and behind where the client's sitting. You're using linguistic markers and voice tones to support the metaphor or example you're using, while you're pacing and leading them. Once you've set this up, then become more direct in your suggestions.

When you're using Conscious-Unconscious Dissociation, you can strengthen that by having two different voice qualities, one for the conscious mind and one for the unconscious mind. I did that with Brantley during his demo. One voice goes to the conscious mind in one location, and another voice to the unconscious mind in another location. After you've done this a few times you've got each one anchored. This is particularly useful because you can utilize these anchors when you're just talking to the client and want to make periodic suggestions outside of a formal trance.

Ecology And Dissociation

It is ecologically important in most cases to **reintegrate whatever you have dissociated.** Generally, you use dissociation to separate something which isn't working optimally as a whole unit. Let's say you have a client who is presenting nightmares as a problem which is secondary to abuse. What is happening is that the effects of the trauma are expressing themselves in the present. Something triggers the recall and the client associates to the trauma. Even though the client is an adult, they will only have whatever resources were available when the original trauma occurred. What you have neurologically is a boundary condition or a "part" which functionally blocks the free flow of information and resources throughout the nervous system. The rationale of using dissociation is that it separates the trauma from the present and temporarily frees the adult from the past trauma. This prevents someone from associating to the "part." This makes it possible to utilize adult resources and understandings to heal the past trauma experienced by the younger self.

After the younger self is healed, you still have one more step to complete. You need to integrate the dissociation so that a new configuration of the whole personality can emerge and take into account the healing of the younger self. If you leave the two selves dissociated, you may have two "healthier parts" but no synergy at the level of personality. There may still be a boundary condition which limits neural transmission. Integrating the two dissolves the neurological boundary condition, the part, and facilitates the free flow of information throughout the nervous system.

Elicitation of Deep Trance Identification (DTI)

Deep Trance Identification is the process whereby you literally assume psychologically, in part or totally, the identity of someone else. This is particularly useful when you find someone who is an exquisite model of something you want. One of the most complete though not universal examples of DTI is Method Acting. What are some other common examples of DTI?

CHRIS: When I speak from the pulpit, I notice I can speak more naturally. When I'm not on the job, I can stutter. When I'm identifying with my job, I don't stutter. Could that be an example?

Sure, because perhaps you identify with being a minister or a professional so when you're doing those activities you do it as they would do it, speaking smoothly and with the flow.

Here's another common example. You're at the movies and you identify with the hero or a particular actor. You feel the fear, the sadness, the excitement, or the joy that they're feeling. One of the main reasons or motivations why people go to the movies is a combination of dissociation and DTI. This has become a billion dollar industry. Movies allow us to escape or dissociate from where we are temporarily, and we can identify with someone who often may be idealized. Notice how many classic, hypnotic phenomena are inverses of one another and/or complementary to each other. As we mentioned in the overview, positive and negative hallucination work this way, as do dissociation and Deep Trance Identification.

Have you ever talked to someone who spoke slowly with pauses in between phrases, or who was a stutterer, and you wanted to finish the sentence for her or him? Have you ever been a passenger in a car and pressed your foot against the floor to brake? If you've ever done this, it was because you were identifying with the driver. That's another everyday example of Deep Trance Identification. Have you ever been around young children and begun to talk "baby talk"? This is actually a combination of DTI and age regression.

Spectator sports also can create DTI. One example, which would be a little too "Neanderthal" for some folks, is boxing; you see the viewers mimicking the micro movements while they're watching. The Cybervision video programs are based on a version of Deep Trance Identification. This producer offers video programs for learning how to ski, play tennis, golf, and lots of other things. They film experts from many angles which make it easy for the viewer to identify with what they're doing. It allows the viewer to practice the micro movements associated with the skill and accelerates learning without actually having to go out and perform the sport. This was a precursor to virtual reality, which may become the lazy person's way to experience Deep Trance Identification in a variety of contexts. Flight simulators would be another example of creating DTI.

Advertising relies heavily on DTI or at least some minimal form of identification. That's why advertisers are willing to pay athletes, musicians, and celebrities large amounts of money. They're hoping that people will identify with the celebrities and buy whatever product the star is wearing or endorsing and imagine that in some way, they'll be like them.

DTI may often be found as a component of the world's great religions. In Christianity, people want to be Christlike. In Buddhism, it's the Buddha. In Hinduism, its Krishna or one of the other incarnations. The idea is to identify with this figure and to embody the positive qualities that the figure or icon represents.

120   TRAINING TRANCES

We can see DTI as a primary process going on behind the scenes in everyday life. As with the other hypnotic skills, our purpose here is to amplify, focus, and refine this skill which we've experienced on a number of levels. Now, for those of you who are going to do DTI in the exercise, whomever you pick as your model, you will need to have specific information about the model with which to identify. The effectiveness of this process is directly proportional to the amount of information you have about that person, which means that you can do it more than once. You can do it here, today, and then later learn more about the person with whom you're identifying. Read books, watch, or listen to tapes; if you can, meet the person directly (or people who have). Obtain as much information as you can, so that's all part of your reference at the unconscious level. This pattern is very generative. Developmentally, it is the basis of some of our earliest and most profound learnings.

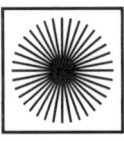

Demonstration of Deep Trance Identification

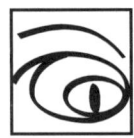

If I were doing Deep Trance Identification with someone, I'd start by making associations. *Now, I know there have been times when you've been at a movie theater and you've been so involved in the movie you could feel exactly how that character was feeling......... Or perhaps you've driven in a car as a passenger and you couldn't help but automatically put your foot on the brake because you identified so closely with the driver.........* (Pacing and leading statements—you add whatever you know about how they have researched the person and what they wanted to replicate.) ..... *I know that you know how to identify in ways that are useful for you to do .... you've done it all your life and you can do it ... Now ....!*

*.... In the same way you can pick someone you want to model ..... I know that there's someone you'd really like to model, to identify with, in a deep way. You've been wanting to identify with this person for some period of time and that person has certain abilities, behaviors, feelings, attitudes that you would really like to begin to experience for yourself. Now, I'm wondering what that person looks like. How would you like to see this person? .... Perhaps at a time when they capture exactly what it is that you want to experience for yourself. It's probably not easy to **imagine** all the information, memories, beliefs, values, and inner workings, just yet ......* (direct suggestion) .. *just looking at that person there .... **Go ahead and see that person** ....*

... And notice that you can easily imagine floating right over into that

person .... Now I don't know when .... you're unconscious .... will make the necessary adjustments to have you float up .... (calibrate).. ..... that's right ..... (higher pitch) up and **float** right (lower pitch) down into this person .... (calibrate to physiological shift) .... so you can begin experiencing the world through the eyes and ears and feelings of this person .... **identify** ..... Now .... I'm not sure how you'll know you're experiencing the world as this person .... only that at the unconscious level we're more similar than we can think about it, and there's a lot more going on at the unconscious level than you can character .... ize ..... seeing, hearing, and feeling ...... being yourself, this person. Now, being this person .... so much to **learn** .... **memorize** it .... so little time to notice consciously what .... who's doing the learning .... that's right, you are, aren't you?

... Perhaps you'll begin to notice, not yet, but when you do, you (your client's name) over there waiting to fully receive what you know now .... go ahead, and as you're ready, **float** right over **into** (your client's model), **yourself** .... (calibrate) .... and allow your unconscious mind to **safely integrate** that information only in a way that is compatible and congruent with and honors your personality, all together, (client's name) you, yourself, **NOW** .... Take all the time you need to allow that integration to complete itself .... **NOW!**

From that point on, if catalepsy occurred, reverse it; bring the client back out and reorient them. You would use your own style of language. The idea is to set up this part of the session with examples of DTI. You have them identify the person and think about what it is about that person they really like. Then they float over into the person, staying there long enough to learn what they want to unconsciously. Then they float back into their body and integrate the information ecologically. A safe suggestion is to float back into your body taking with you only that which is valuable to you or in your best interest. That's the DTI pattern.

Ecology And Deep Trance Identification

Although DTI is naturally occurring, like other classical hypnotic phenomena, there are a few matters to consider when you use it purposely with yourself or a client. When you're working with someone, it's generally a good idea to know up front with whom they're choosing to identify. You want the person to consider the ramifications of identifying with the model. As a safeguard, you can always tell the unconscious mind—as you begin and at any point along the way—that it can disregard any suggestions that you make that aren't in its best interests. **Your unconscious mind always has the ability to know the difference between suggestions which are good for it and suggestions which aren't.** If you really want to check it out, ask, "You do understand that, don't you?" Get a "yes." It's a nice general suggestion which you can put in at any time in any of your hypnosis sessions.

Since a fair amount of dissociation is needed to facilitate the Deep Trance Identification with the model, remember to take into account all that you learned when doing dissociation: **integrate, integrate, integrate.** You can use this pattern to do remedial work or you can use it proactively for generative results. Depending on your intention, DTI can be a fast, handy kind of pattern (when you leave out the "deep trance") to assist someone in creating a resource which they can't locate in their own personal history. The real power of this skill blossoms during deep trance. When done with care and consideration of personal ecology, it truly is a trans-formation-al(l) way to create change.

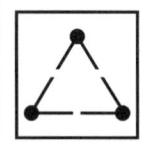

Elicitation And Utilization of Hypnotic Phenomena Exercise

1. Induce trance.
2. Elicit catalepsy and deepen trance.
3. Elicit selected hypnotic phenomena:
    a. provide universal examples to activate the appropriate neural networks.
    b. pace and lead the client's current experience toward the desired response. (This serves as the bridge between the associations activated in a. and the direct suggestion in c.)
    c. directly suggest the desired response only after you have sensory verification of its development.
4. Give suggestion to thoroughly memorize the skill.
    a. check ecology.
    b. calibrate to agreement. You can use "yes/no" signals if you want.
5. Posthypnotic Suggestion:
"Identify where in the future you want to manifest this ability and play it through as many times as you'd like to fully appreciate your ability to learn new things that can help you and others."

Uh, oh! Don just fastened his seat belt.

We're still building. This will be fun. Remember, what are the three things you know about the person sitting across from you?

AUDIENCE: **You're a great hypnotic subject. You're totally resourceful. You change easily and timely.**

That's right . . . . and remember they've already experienced the hypnotic phenomena, which you're going to assist them with in this exercise, many times in their everyday lives. The most you'll be doing is helping them to expand and amplify what they already know how to do. Let's take fifteen minutes per person—make sure that you have time to set up the associations so everything flows smoothly.

Do the exercise

Discussion

CINDY: I experienced total body analgesia and I hadn't planned to. My conscious attention was so narrowly focused on my neck that the sensations in my neck became the trance induction.

That's great, because you were so focused on your neck that you weren't paying attention to all their other suggestions for full body analgesia. You had a direct experience of what we were referring to earlier. Let your clients choose where to fixate their attention and make that the basis of your induction.

TEMPA: I noticed I had spontaneous amnesia for the induction.

That's right, we keep forgetting to cover that. Actually, we decided to wait to give you a formal procedure for eliciting amnesia, because it's so easy to generate it spontaneously. The easiest way to create amnesia is to have a person go in and out of deep trance a number of times. It's just that simple because of the way our neurology is set up. Since trance states are so separate from normal waking states, it's too wide of a discrepancy in the levels of awareness. It's similar to comparing dreaming to the waking state. It is not easy to bring back all the information from our dreams; and it's useful to have a natural amnesia like this, because it is created by the unconscious mind to support the ecology of change.

124   TRAINING TRANCES

AUDIENCE: Could you give us a rough estimate of how much time it takes to produce certain hypnotic phenomena? How long do you work to elicit a certain one, before you look for other alternatives?

You take whatever time is necessary for your client to get the results. That takes the pressure off you and off your client. You base it upon how quickly you and your client can move together. Some people can produce a hypnotic phenomenon spontaneously, while others like to develop it gradually. It's a lot like trance. We've heard that when Erickson was asked if he had ever not succeeded in hypnotizing a subject, he answered (paraphrasing), "No, and there are still a few that I'm still working with." Ultimately, the only thing that would prevent a hypnotherapist from producing certain hypnotic phenomena would be putting time limits on the development of it.

Therefore, sometimes you may train your clients in doing trance and catalepsy for several sessions before doing the analgesia—which may have been the actual outcome of the therapy. In other cases, some people come in and produce analgesia in an hour without even lifting a finger. It just depends on the person with whom you're working—so you always tailor your work to whomever is sitting in front of you. That's the most respectful way and also the easiest. There's that old question of how long does it take for a person to change? It takes as long as it takes.

DAVE: How do you know which hypnotic skill to use when there may be several that could work? Like with pain control, we could use dissociation, analgesia, or anesthesia.

Let's say your client has seen a doctor and has a prescription to see you. You interview the client, find out about the symptom, the possible psychological function of the symptom, and elicit a well-formed outcome. While you're collecting this information, you might also *be curious* about times when they don't have the symptom. What are they doing or not doing in these situations? Listen carefully to what they do naturally, outside of their awareness, which may be associated with times when they don't have the symptom. *Pay attention* to casual remarks they make that tip you off to hypnotic skills they're already using in other areas of their life. Remember, as you're looking for the skills, you'll usually have your best success when they're not talking about the symptom. Most of the time, your client's unconscious mind will make sure they tell you exactly what you need to know to assist them. As you hear and notice these things, they will help you decide which hypnotic skills will be the most appropriate, as well as the means for producing them. More than the "techniques," it is this sort of observation which made Erickson so effective. His techniques grew naturally from his observations. Many of us have wondered how Milton could have been privy to so many nuances in others' experiences. We'll give you a hint: he didn't do it with his conscious mind. He was always willing to trust his unconscious mind. Right up to his death, he continued to use many of the same experiential understandings, learnings, and hypnotic skills which he helped so many others *develop fully* in themselves. It's inspiring to consider that a farm boy from the Midwest accomplished so much and touched so many during his lifetime—and after—considering all of his seeming limitations. The world could use a few more like him. Milton was willing to use what he had. He was willing to *trust* that he was much more than he thought he was. Just consider what can happen when *you do that*.

Chapter 7

The Hypnotic Interview: The Inner View of Trans-Formation

Editor's Notes: Erickson rarely made explicit process comments about his work. He taught in much the same way he did therapy—indirectly. Therefore, in this chapter, the trainers use several of Erickson's more well-known cases to identify and codify the common elements found in his hypnotherapy sessions. The structure of the chapter mirrors the structure of the hypnotic interview itself. As an aside, the trainers are unaware of any other written work which details the steps of Dr. Erickson's hypnotic interview and the thought processes instrumental in its development (see Reframing). Their intention with this format is to assist the reader in understanding and beginning to replicate Erickson's work.

Question to the reader: How did Erickson devise the treatment plan or the theme for the therapy?

This section is about integrating the material which was covered in the previous chapters. As we do that, it's important to underscore that the particular structure of an interview is as varied as the hypnotherapist who conducts it. In our study of documented Erickson interviews, there are definite commonalities in his approaches, although it is obvious that he did whatever he needed to do to assist a patient in moving from point A to point B. The following is one structure which we modeled for this Training in Trance because it is easy to teach and to understand, and it is generic enough to use in most therapy sessions. You'll recognize this format for the hypnotic interview because we've done exercises which utilized its component parts.

In fact, perhaps you've noticed that this training has been taught in the sequence in which you would be using many of these skills during a therapeutic interview. If you have, this is another good indication that you're learning far more at the unconscious level than you could know consciously. It can be comforting to know that unconscious learning always precedes conscious recognition. It's not immediately important that you verify this in other areas of your life for the purposes of your learning here, because we don't know what new patterns you'll recognize later that may serve as even better examples. This particular model of the hypnotic interview gives you enough structure to know where you are and where you need to go, yet it leaves plenty of room to improvise based upon your client's responses.

Overview of The Hypnotic Interview

1. Elicitation of the Problem State and Desired (Outcome) State

2. Conscious-Unconscious Dissociation

3. Utilization of Hypnotic Phenomena

4. Changework

5. Posthypnotic Suggestion

6. Reorientation and Distraction of Conscious Attention

To encapsulate the structure of this interview, a problem state and an outcome state are elicited. Then the problem is temporarily associated to the conscious mind and the resources are associated to the unconscious mind. This step is used as a vehicle to induce trance via Conscious-Unconscious Dissociation. In Step 3, trance is deepened through the utilization of Hypnotic Phenomena. This is followed by the changework section, where one major reframe is created by separating behavior (or sensation or symptom) from intention. This reframe becomes the theme of the therapy session. Then, the client engages in an unconscious search to revivify resources. Analogy or metaphor may be used at this point to support the reframe and the outcome. The interview concludes with posthypnotic suggestion and reorientation. There will be an expanded posthypnotic protocol in a later section modeled from Erickson's work. For this interview model, the posthypnotic suggestion is a shortened version with two components: one using direct suggestion and one using indirect suggestion.

Milton's Inner View—Before The Interview

This section is designed to assist you in considering the thought processes you would go through before you do this type of work. In the clinical setting, you'll obtain whatever background information you deem necessary. Listening to "content" is often a balancing act between the client's need to disclose pertinent information and the therapist's desire for just enough material to understand the structure of the problem. While the content may provide you with the information necessary to make a traditional diagnosis, that same content may pull you into the client's problem "trance," particularly if you're looking for the answer within the content. To the extent that you're in an outside (uptime) trance and oriented toward their unconscious communication, you'll know if and when to elicit more content.

Theoretically, you could do this entire intervention content-free, calibrating only to your client's nonverbal responses. You could say, "You've had a problem and it's something you've wanted to change for some time now. (Calibrating to whether you have agreement or not.) And you know there is a certain outcome or outcomes that are of interest to you, correct?" Now you're just talking about problems and outcomes and you can keep it on that level and never chunk down to the specifics of their particular problem. Sometimes it is useful to chunk down to determine what the problem and outcome are, so that you can observe the nonverbal analogs associated with their descriptions of each. Having these specifics determines which words will activate the necessary neural networks associated with the problem and the outcome. Also, gathering some details will pace most clients' expectations that therapy is talking about their problems.

Erickson would often spend a considerable amount of time getting a history from a person. This interestingly is the haziest area of his work because he talked very little about how he gathered information. A number of case studies shed some light on his subtle utilization of clients' memories, reveries, and state changes during the information-gathering process.[1] We've never read or seen anyone discuss at any length exactly how he structured this part of therapy, although we do know that he was very interested in clients' values.[2] This is how he often motivated his clients to carry out seemingly outrageous tasks for the resolution of their problems. Since we don't have a substantial amount of information on Erickson regarding this area, we will rely on the NLP notion of problem and outcome states.

Our impression is that, depending on the case, Erickson might inquire about all the typical things which therapists ask: family history, medical history, employment history, and past history of the problem (all of the standard information which would be part of an intake process). Quite often he also asked about people's personal interests. What did they like to do? What were their hobbies? In what areas did they naturally excel? Casually talking to clients about their interests can be a very disarming and effective way to identify and revivify their internal resources, while providing preliminary ideas about which metaphors will be most suitable for the therapy. As discussed earlier, this is an area of the interview where it is beneficial to chunk down, because eliciting specifics will intensify the state and enable the therapist to anchor these states for later use. Additionally, most people enjoy talking about their interests and hobbies, and while they are doing that, the therapist has the opportunity to begin laying the groundwork of the intervention, so it flows easily and resonates with the client at a deep level.

For example: Julie loves skiing. If you were working with Julie, you could begin by having her talk about skiing; revivifying confidence, excitement, and pleasure; and later even using skiing as a metaphor to support a therapeutic theme. The process for resolving the presenting problem could be likened in some way to the process of skiing. This will fully engage her conscious mind while activating various resources at the unconscious level. It then also becomes the backdrop for interspersing embedded commands and other generative suggestions.

Eliciting skills and resources from the client's personal history and from contexts which are unrelated to the client's presenting problem is the best approach. If you watch the Monde tape, you'll see Erickson regress Monde to a time when she was quite young and was "splashing in the water"[3] and "chasing ducks."[4] Erickson anchors this state and then chains it to a series of other early experiences. Any experience within the client's personal history is a possibility for resource elicitation—including going into the future.

In one case, Erickson induced trance and oriented his client to a point in the future where the client was seeing Erickson for a follow-up interview and discussing how much he had changed![5] Erickson asked the client about the aspects of therapy which were the most effective; what was done in each session; and how many sessions it entailed. Erickson took copious notes on all this information and then reoriented the client after providing multiple suggestions for amnesia. He then scheduled another appointment and dismissed the client. How did he know what to do in the next session? He simply followed the entire treatment plan which was designed by the client's unconscious mind. All Erickson had to do was follow the instructions!

The idea of future projection has been utilized for years. Another way which isn't as dramatic, but which is very empowering, is to have the client carry on a conversation with the future self who has successfully gone beyond the current problem. This dialogue activates a wonderful archetype: the older, wiser self. What advice does the future self have for them? What did they do?

What did they learn that made the difference? The key to making this work is to ensure that the clients are effectively dissociated and disoriented from the present. Otherwise, when they consult their future self—and we've run into this—they'll say, "I don't know what I did," and then collapse back into the presenting problem. Layering trance states to create amnesia will create greater dissociation and often lessen the likelihood of reassociating to the problem.

Gathering information in this way, from areas of interest or from resources, both past and future, is unique. The value of this technique is not only in the information gathered, but perhaps even more importantly, in repeatedly conditioning the client to trance, without any direct mention of trance. In some cases the presenting issue can be quickly resolved by asking questions which activate and intensify the states necessary for achieving the outcome. However, if eliciting these resources does not resolve the problem, it's all right because technically the "changework" has not been done yet. The hypnotherapist was just gathering information.

The Hypnotic Interview

Step 1: Elicitation of problem state and desired (outcome) state exercise

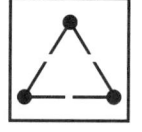

1. Elicit problem state. "What are you doing or feeling that you want to change?"
2. Break rapport after eliciting the problem state:
   a. change voice tone.
   b. change physiology.
3. Elicit outcome: "What do you want?" ("How do you want to be feeling or behaving instead?")
   a. positively stated.
   b. succinct.
   *c. optional: If you know the NLP outcome frame questions and well-formedness conditions, use them. (See Appendix.)
4. Check congruency and ecology:
   a. repeat client's statement of outcome, "What you want is . . ."
   b. make sure all components of communication (physiology, voice tone and words) are aligned and symmetrical.

Find a new partner and elicit a problem and an outcome. Ask your partner to pick something small—unless they're a mismatcher (one who always does the opposite) and then they should pick the biggest issue of their life. Also pick something which they will be able to verify for themselves once the change has taken place. A good choice would generally be a problem which involves a change of state in a specific context. Is there a situation (or a set of situations) where your partner has a certain feeling they don't like and which they want to change? The purpose of this exercise is to practice this format rather than to create transformation. *You can do all that on your own quite well.* Write this information down because it will be useful during the next few steps. Ready, go!

Do the exercise

Step 2: Conscious-Unconscious Dissociation: some truth about solving problems

If you want to use this interview structure with minimal content, it would be useful to add these truisms about problems. Doing so will give you a chance to create a "yes" set and establish rapport without delving into content. In fact, the client only needs to respond nonverbally and all you're doing is calibrating to agreement. Even if you were using content during the interview, these truisms are still very useful for the same reasons.

When you deliver these statements, it's important to do so with the same kind of caring and compassion you would if you knew what the content was. Many therapists unconsciously rely on the content to inspire the resources of caring and compassion in themselves. Content is not necessary for doing this. Additionally, if you have analogically marked words or phrases which the client offered during the problem and outcome elicitation, you can incorporate these with the truisms.

(Trainer begins reading the list.) *"You've had this problem for some time. It's made your life more difficult than you want and you've tried to resolve it on your own more than once. When you really think about it, it's affected other areas in your life and you haven't been able to **know what you can do.**"*

You might wonder if this isn't installing more problems, so it may be worthwhile to consider the following. Truisms work in a presuppositional way, because if they answer "yes" to the above and later make a change, what's implied is that the change will generalize to other areas of their life. So you trade one for the other. You have to emphasize "really." "Really" is a very important word hypnotically. When you emphasize it, it causes the listener to reconsider what is being said in a different way. For example, "Think about it

..... no, really think about it." Notice the difference between the two? "Really" makes you consider it more deeply.

*"It's something you can no longer ignore or put off without getting more of the same. If the **time to change** isn't now, it's soon approaching. You've wondered if you can really **change this** .... if it's really possible. And you've not been able to fully **succeed at overcoming it**. You may wonder what **you can begin now** ... to change this."*

Truisms allow you to talk about what the client is experiencing without going too deeply into a "content trance." They are also useful because they anchor the problem state and they include a number of important presuppositions which will be utilized later in the interview.

Truisms About Solving Problems

You've had this problem for some time . . .
It has made your life more difficult than you want . . .
You have tried to resolve it on your own more than once . . .
In fact, you've spent more time thinking about it than you'd like . . .
When you really think about it, it has affected other areas of your life . . .
And you haven't been able to **know what you can do** . . .
But you do know it is something that you can no longer ignore or put off without getting more of what you don't want . . .
If the **time to change** isn't **NOW**, it's soon approaching . . .
Until now you have wondered if you can really **change this**, if it's really possible . . .
And even though you've not been able to fully **succeed at overcoming it** . . .
You may wonder what **you can begin NOW to change.**

You then anchor the problem state to the conscious mind and anchor the outcome to the unconscious mind. And, yes, this is just a metaphor. It's not entirely true, but it creates more possibilities when the unconscious is everything else other than the problem. It's more likely that your unconscious has the solution, because if it were conscious, you would have already known what the solution was and would have implemented it. As with the standard Conscious-Unconscious Dissociation induction, you'll use voice tone and locus anchors to further stabilize the dissociation.

Group Demonstration

Consciously, you've <u>tried</u> to resolve this issue on your own, while your unconscious mind knows what the root of the problem <u>really</u> is. And while you've consciously spent more time thinking about this problem than you'd like, your unconscious mind has been thinking about more important things. Your conscious mind can only attend to a very limited amount of information . . .

. . . while your unconscious has recorded all of your experiences. It's the storehouse of all of your memories. Everything you've ever seen, everything you've ever heard, everything you've ever felt, smelled, tasted, and said to yourself is recorded at the unconscious level. So, consciously you may be wondering how **you can change** this, because it's your unconscious mind that knows how to change and **do it timely and easily**. Whether or not you consciously think you know what to do, it's your unconscious mind that can begin considering what's <u>really</u> important to you and **begin finding resources**, not necessarily to change, **NOW**, but to make this an experience that will serve as a foundation for your learning how to **go into a trance**, **NOW** . . .

. . . . because consciously, you may not fully recognize that you are in a trance, because your conscious mind may be focusing on other things; perhaps you're aware of the sounds in the room, sensations in your body, your increasing comfort or perhaps something else more interesting to you, while listening to me . . . .

You'll do the same Conscious-Unconscious Dissociation induction which you did earlier; you're just layering in the problem and solution. Next you'll elicit and utilize the hypnotic phenomena which will serve as resources to move the client to the outcome.

Step 3: Utilization of hypnotic phenomena: deepen the trance, communicate directly with the unconscious, and activate the hypnotic skills

We've labeled the third step in the hypnotic interview as utilizing hypnotic phenomena. Utilization of hypnotic phenomena and/or ideomotor responses can assist the hypnotherapist in deepening the trance, establishing direct communication with the unconscious mind ("yes" and "no" signals), and formulating resources. Erickson frequently used catalepsy as the basic hypnotic phenomenon, from which the others derived. We will also use catalepsy as our primary resource in this section.

What is valuable about catalepsy is that it creates another predictable kind of event inside trance with which you can coordinate the client's responses. As discussed in the previous chapter, catalepsy is useful as a gauge. It's a gross gauge of whether the person is in trance and at about what level they are. They're in a medium level trance if they display catalepsy. They may be on either side of "medium" on the continuum (a light trance moving into a medium one or a medium moving to a deeper one). Catalepsy is also an analog gauge which you can use to indicate how far along a client's unconscious mind is in completing a suggested task. Typical ideomotor signals are digital (either "yes" or "no"), not analog, and consequently provide only a limited amount of information.

Take this suggestion as an example: "I don't want that hand to go down only as quickly as you find all those resources." You'll know where the client is in the process by where the levitating arm is in relation to the leg. If it's moving and then stops at the halfway point for a period of time, that's a good indication that you need to check in and find out what's going on. If you have additional tasks you want to suggest and monitor, you can continue to bring the hand back up for each of the tasks. It's a lot like hourglass timers used in cooking. This way you'll know when the change is well done.

You have another predictable opportunity because you know the hand is going to return to their lap. You can anchor suggestions to that: *". . . And as that hand rests fully on your lap, you may notice a feeling of warmth . . . . that can begin to spread . . . throughout your body . . . that may remind you of those resources spreading throughout the areas of your life which will support your total integration . . ."*

Step 4. Changework into new unconscious possibilities
    a. reframe the intention
    b. create the theme for the transformation
    c. begin unconscious search to activate resources

a. Reframe the intention

There are literally thousands of approaches for doing "changework." There are many choices available for the hypnotherapist who has been trained in NLP. Reframing is emphasized because it was part of the standard interview which we modeled from Dr. Erickson's work.[6,7,8]

A reframe is simply a different point of view which, in its best therapeutic application, expands possibilities. Neurologically, it stimulates additional neural networks which can collapse, or at least diminish, the boundary conditions of the neural networks associated with the problem. The central feature in the construction of a reframe is the separation of behavior from intention. All meaning is context dependent. Therefore the only way to evaluate anything, be it an idea or concept, a word or series of words, a sensation or feeling, or a behavior or activity, is to consider the context in which it occurs. What may work in one context may not work in another.

The behaviors, feelings, or symptoms which bring most clients into therapy have served some positive function for them at another point or within another context in their life. We believe this from a spiritual point of view and also from the biological point of view of survival. There's a positive intent behind every behavior no matter how maladaptive it is. This doesn't mean the behavior is acceptable, because it may be something which is very dysfunctional, but there will be a positive intention behind it.

To elicit the highest intention of the problem, you simply ask the unconscious mind, "What is your highest intention in (state the <u>problem</u>)?" Another choice is to "mind read" what the highest intention of the problem would be instead of directly asking the client. This information will be valuable when the theme for the therapy is established.

AUDIENCE:
> Could you elaborate a bit more on the "chunking up to the highest positive intention?"

Certainly. First, let's discuss the purpose for considering the highest positive intention of the problem. Identifying the highest intention tends to prevent symptom substitution or secondary gain. By preserving the highest intention of the problem behavior or state, you're increasing the integrity of the total personality. You're saying, "Your intention is good. Let's find other ways which will satisfy your intention and increase congruency and choice."

As mentioned above, one option is for you to ask the client directly the highest intention of the problem when you elicit the problem. Your second option is to mind read what their intention might be and utilize that. (See the Appendix for basic reframing structures.) No matter how you arrive at the highest intention of the problem, you want to make sure that it is represented as a state. You will need to chunk up high enough to reach an abstraction which is an emotion. This is the state you will then revivify as we go through the changework section.

Since you already know the client's problem and outcome, you may have already arrived at the theme you're going to use for the therapy. If you haven't yet elicited the highest intention for the behavior, here are some questions you can ask yourself about the client to accomplish this.

> ## Mind Reading Positive Intention
>
> "What positive intention could account for the underlying motivation of the unwanted behavior?"
>
> "What positive value could this have?"
>
> "What is this symptom or behavior an example of?"

The information gathered as you reframed the problem sets up the theme for therapeutic transformation, which is the next step.

b. Create the theme for transformation

Now that you have elicited the problem and the outcome state and have reframed the problem, you can begin to make some decisions about which themes will be included in the interview. The theme then becomes the basis of your working "treatment plan." While working with your client you can adjust this based upon their responses and your sensory acuity.

To create the theme, you first determine the "hidden ability" which the problem and outcome have in common. Believe it or not, each problem and outcome presuppose common traits. Discovering these common hidden abilities will guide you toward the metaphors and universals which will be most effective in the therapy. Your goal will be to light up parallel neural networks and associations, to demonstrate how the common hidden ability can be used in a positive way, consistent with the outcome. The questions to ask yourself to determine these commonalities are in the box on the next page.

> **Uncovering Hidden Common Abilities**
>
> "What positive abilities, skills, or resources are, or could be inherent in the problem and the outcome?"
>
> "In order to do this problem, what must she/he be good at?"
>
> "What context or where would this problem actually be worthwhile?"
>
> "What hypnotic skill is presupposed in both?"

There are some universals for most problems. For example, if a person has a chronic problem, you know for sure that inherent in chronicity is persistence and tenacity. If they have pain, then they already understand trance. If they are paranoid, we know they excel at positive hallucination. Remember, behavior is only a problem to the extent it doesn't fit the context where it's occurring.

So let's use a problem that was presented during the exercise as an example of one way to do this.

MARILYN:
>My problem is I don't read fast enough. I used to be able to read very quickly (voice begins to quiver and eyes begin to tear) . . . . I guess I made a decision . . . . Now, I control the speed it comes in and subvocalize . . . . It happened in school. I was reading and made a mistake and the teacher made an example of me in front of the whole class. I guess I've never quite gotten over it . . . . (takes a deep breath, voice becomes steadier) . . . I want to read fast again and remember what I read.

This is summarized on the next page.

Developing The Reframe And Theme For Transformation

Problem: Reads slowly—subvocalizes when reading.

Outcome: Read fast with comprehension.

Intention as presented: To not make mistakes and to not get into trouble.

Highest intention: Relax and enjoy learning.

As she chunked up to higher levels of abstraction, the intention of not making mistakes and getting in trouble was to "please the teacher." If she could please the teacher, she would get "approval." If she had "approval," she could "relax and enjoy learning." It's important to reach a logical level that is represented as a state that is the <u>opposite</u> of the problem. This will give you leverage at the unconscious level to make the change.

Common abilities:
1. She can **control** the speed. (She stated that now she controls the speed and subvocalizes. The fact that she can slow it down presupposes that she can speed it up.)

2. She can **make decisions** very quickly and **generalize** them to other areas of her life. (She said she made a "decision" that essentially reading fast meant she might make a mistake and get into trouble. This "decision" was in response to criticism by a teacher.)

Theme for transformation:
(Use indirect suggestions for lighter trance or to set up direct suggestions.)
1. *A long time ago, you had to decide to slow down the speed of your reading. You learned you can control the speed of your reading . . . NOW . . . How much faster will you find yourself reading and remembering what you've read having decided to relax and enjoy learning?*

> Continued...
>
> (Use direct suggestions stated permissively for deeper trance.)
>
> 2. *You can make decisions quickly and generalize them. You can decide to read faster. You can control the speed of your reading. You can read fast and remember what you've read. You can relax and enjoy learning.*

Another fascinating example comes directly from *Hypnotherapy: An Exploratory Casebook* by Erickson and Rossi. It relates to a session Erickson had with an older man who had phantom limb pain and his wife who had tinnitus.[9] One of Erickson's primary reframes for the phantom limb pain was, "If you can feel phantom pain, you can feel phantom pleasure." That's a context reframe. We don't really know what Erickson's thought processes were at the time, but one way to reframe pain into pleasure is to ask, "What ability does the person have, to be able to feel pain in a part of their body that doesn't exist anymore?" The answer is positive (tactile) hallucination, which is the ability to create and experience sensations outside the physical body. This ability is then utilized as a resource to achieve the outcome of pain reduction, or restated in the positive, to achieve "pleasure."

Constructing the reframe breaks up the constellation of the problem while highlighting heretofore hidden abilities. Strategically, it creates the overall theme for the therapy and the transformation: if the client can create phantom pain, then he/she can create phantom pleasure. The reframed ability is linked to common hypnotic phenomena, automatic processes, emotional states, and life experiences which are activated when the client's in trance. The metaphors which are used will be based upon the theme and the inherent abilities which were identified.

c. Begin unconscious search to activate resources

In this phase of the changework, you will be activating associations that will flesh out and support the reframe(s) developed previously. This is where the client's vast unconscious resources are activated, reorganized, and aligned with the desired outcome.

In the phantom pain example, the inherent ability which is operating is positive hallucination. To facilitate the unconscious search, you start to talk about everyday examples of positive hallucination to activate the appropriate neural networks. After you activate the associations, then directly suggest the hypnotic phenomena with the reframe. "Therefore, if you've felt phantom pain, you can feel phantom pleasure." What is wonderful about working this way is that you don't try to solve the problem for the client. You, as the hypnotherapist, can't solve the problem anyhow: it's up to the client. What you are doing is creating an optimal context for change via hypnosis so what is being suggested is fully considered by the client's unconscious mind. Hypnosis is an inner-directed state where one pays attention to what is immediately important and deletes the irrelevancies. Once in trance, you are just facilitating the activation of latent resources which had been previously overlooked.

One way to think about this is to consider that everything we've ever seen, heard, felt, smelled, tasted, and said to ourselves has been recorded at the unconscious level. Our experiences are stored as memories. Each memory has within it pieces which make up that particular memory, i.e. what we saw, what we heard, what sensations we felt, what emotions we experienced, what we said to ourselves, our movements, our behaviors, and our internal resources. All of these comprise the raw data of our memories and experiences.

*"Wouldn't it be interesting to consider that **your unconscious** mind could perhaps take one tiny piece of one memory; maybe something you felt, and combine it with a piece from another memory; maybe something you thought, and combine those with a piece from another memory, maybe something you said and it could continue combining these pieces to **create a totally new way of learning** that would be in complete alignment with the highest intentions of your personality. In fact your unconscious mind puts pieces together like this all the time, for instance, as you sleep and dream . . . . **Now** . . . . I don't know how many new behaviors to **increase your learning** your unconscious mind can generate, perhaps as few as five or many more. I do know that it's not important that your conscious mind knows what the new ways to learn are because it didn't generate any of the old ones anyway. Your conscious mind might like to think it knows one or two of the new behaviors, while your unconscious . . . . . . generates new ways to learn outside of your awareness. And your conscious mind will know that your unconscious mind has, in fact, completed this search by giving you a signal, so your conscious mind nose it's just beginning to scratch the surface unconsciously."*

Step 5. The posthypnotic suggestion: suggest trance directly and change, by presupposition

In this short version of the posthypnotic suggestion structure, all that is directly suggested is, "You *will be able to go into trance easily the next time*

. . . anytime thereafter you want to do it." Now just think about this. Why would you, the hypnotherapist, want to suggest something this general if your client was there for a specific reason? Here's a hint: what state is your client in when they do the changework? TRANCE. What do you think will happen when they access trance the next time as you've suggested? They will be entering that same state. And what will they find there? The work you've just done with them. They're going to find that file (state) when they access the folder (trance). Every time they participate in this, they are revivifying and reinforcing what occurred inside of trance, which is really neat! Even though it's a direct suggestion for trance, it's totally indirect relative to the outcome. It suggests the outcome by presupposition because they're going to be revivifying the process involved in achieving it.

In the indirect component, you'll future pace them by presupposition. *"I don't know when you're going to know you've changed. Maybe it will be tomorrow, maybe it will be the next day, or perhaps just after you wake up, who knows? . . . . . . And I don't know how you're going to notice it—will it be something that comes to you in a sudden insight or will you notice it more gradually?"* These are some quick examples. You can wonder or ask all sorts of things out loud to your client which will presuppose the outcome. Use interrogatives such as how, when, and where. However, if they're deeply in trance, then just directly suggest that the next time you see/hear (stimulus) you're going to (outcome).

Step 6. Reorient and distract: "Welcome back" and "It's nice outside today, isn't?"

You finish by reorienting your clients and distracting their conscious attention. Why would you want to do that? This is another way of sealing off the work you've done. It's another way of creating partial or full amnesia, depending on what kind of trancework you were doing. You might say, "Hi, how are you doing?" and then start talking about anything other than what you just did with them.

One of the classic temptations for me after doing changework is to interview the person about all the great things that happened. That's ego. Let it go. Later, like the next time they come in, if they want to discuss it, that's fine. One of the only times to discuss what occurred in trance is when the trance is being reinduced. Asking them about the previous hypnotic experience can be used to elicit trance. We demonstrated that with a couple of the induction demos we did. If the person is reentering trance for some purpose, the easiest way to do that is to start asking them very detailed questions about the trance. What do they have to do to answer those questions? They have to go back into the state to retrieve the information.

TEMPA: Should we always distract conscious attention after we've finished the trancework?

It depends on your outcome. Generally, if you're finished, then distract their conscious attention. If you're just conditioning trance and educating your client about the experience of hypnosis, though, you might want to ask them about the physical sensations in their body to verify the trance experience for them. Whether or not you distract conscious attention is largely contingent upon what you know about your client. Will conscious validation contribute to the success of the work or not? Sometimes a mixed understanding is useful; that is, conscious validation that trance or a shift of some type occurred but amnesia for the actual therapeutic work which transpired. This often happens naturally, particularly if you've induced a series of trances throughout the session.

The primary reason why Erickson used amnesia is because it protects the work that's been done from conscious interference on the client's part.[10] This is important for people who are highly intellectualized about their problems or people who have been heavily conditioned to content-oriented therapy and have not experienced a change. Some clients, after a therapy session which went well, spend the next intervening period of time trying to figure out when the changes they made won't work! Amnesia makes the therapeutic information unavailable for analysis until such time as they've made the change. Then it generally bubbles up into their awareness because they recognize that they're doing something differently.

Also, this doesn't mean they have to have complete amnesia for the hypnotherapy to have been successful. They might remember some of what was said and they may have forgotten the rest because in trance they only pay attention to what is immediately important and the rest just goes into the unconscious mind.

One way to induce amnesia before starting the induction is to ask a question and not follow through with any discussion of it. Ask, for example, "Meredith, where are you headed after you leave here today?" and then just move on. She may or may not answer it. When she comes out of trance you ask the same question, "Meredith, where did you say you were going after you leave here today?" So ask a question at the beginning, do the entire hypnotic interview, and ask the identical question after they've come out of trance. This often has the effect of sending one back in time to when it was previously asked. There are many variations to this method, depending on how the topic which was introduced at the beginning of the session is resumed.

Erickson would take what we're discussing here a step further. At the beginning of a session, he would go halfway into a sentence or an idea and stop and then at the end pick up as if he never stopped. You ask, "Meredith, where are you going after this?" Meredith replies, "Home." Then you do the trance induction .... (to Meredith), "And where is it you're going home to?"

With this one, you have to remember exactly where you were. It's usually easy to remember the general category of the question you were asking. The critical component of inducing amnesia this way is to remember the state you were in when you were asking the question. This often will be more important than repeating the same question or picking up where you left off. When you revivify the state you were in and resume the same conversation, it will likely revivify the state the client was in at the beginning of the session. Doing this adroitly can create a very interesting a déjà vu experience, which surrounds the actual trance experience, and if that doesn't create amnesia, nothing will! Using some variation of this approach is generally an easier way to create amnesia than suggesting it directly. Other direct ways of suggesting trance will be discussed later in the posthypnotic suggestion section.

Setup For The Exercise

You will begin with Conscious-Unconscious Dissociation first, thus dissociating the problem from the outcome. The next step is to utilize one of the hypnotic phenomena (most likely catalepsy) to deepen the trance. Then you'll deliver your reframe or a number of reframes for that matter. After this, the unconscious search begins, as you invite your partner to go through their personal history to locate experiences which support the reframe. When they do this, they are building a generalization or a belief.

As you revivify these experiences, you can link these with the hypnotic phenomena. The way you do that is to create associations first, and then you directly suggest what you want them to do, and then you connect that to the problem. The final piece before reorientation is the posthypnotic suggestion. Here you suggest directly that they'll be able to go into trance easily whenever they want and where it's appropriate. The indirect suggestion is, "I don't know just how quickly you'll make this change. Or when you'll make it. Only that you'll have a growing sense of anticipation of how good it will feel to have made the change." Then assist them in reorienting and ask something such as, "What did you say the weather prediction for the weekend was?" The complete interview is illustrated in Figure 7.1 on the next page.

The Hypnotic Interview: The Inner View of Trans-Formation   145

ELICITATION OF
PRESENT STATE
& OUTCOME

INDUCTION

- Pacing
- Revivification
- Conscious-unconscious Dissociation

UTILIZATION
OF HYPNOTIC
PHENOMENA

- Ideomotor signals
- Catalepsy
- Other hypnotic skills

CHANGEWORK
- Reframe intentions
- Unconscious search to activate resources
- Create theme for Transformation

POSTHYPNOTIC SUGGESTION
- Indirectly suggest desired outcome
- Directly suggest trance

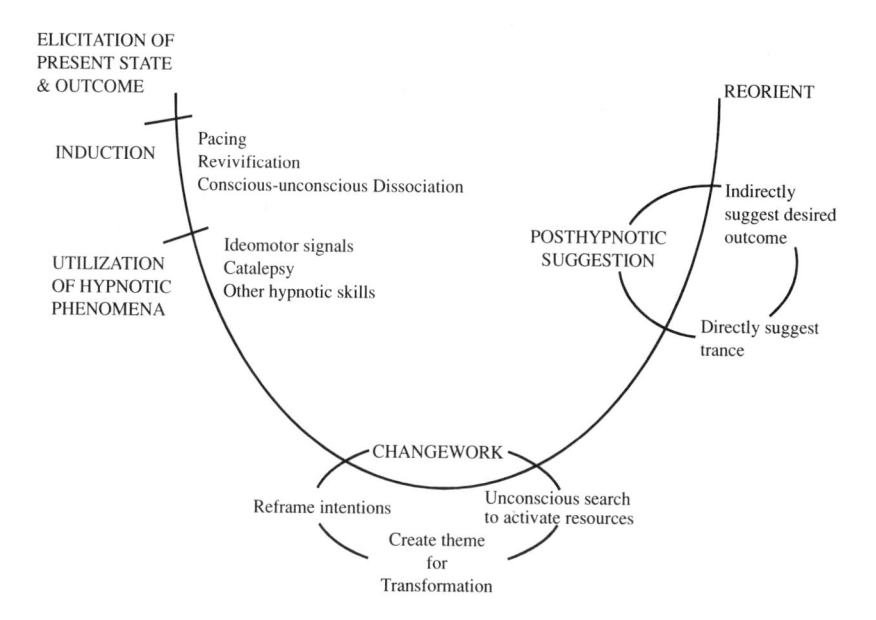

REORIENT

Figure 7.1
The Hypnotic Interview

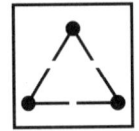

The Hypnotic Interview Exercise

1. Elicitation of the problem and desired state.

2. Conscious-Unconscious Dissociation:
   a. dissociate conscious from unconscious.
   b. anchor problem to conscious mind and solution to unconscious mind.

3. Utilization of hypnotic phenomena:
   a. to deepen trance.
   b. set up direct communication with the unconscious mind.
   c. begin activating resources which support the changework.

4. Changework into new unconscious possibilities:
   a. reframe the intention.
   b. create the theme for the transformation.
   c. begin unconscious search to activate resources.

5. Posthypnotic suggestion:
   a. direct—able to go into trance easily.
   b. indirect—presupposes outcome.

6. Reorientation and distraction of conscious attention.

Do the exercise

This protocol for a hypnotic interview, in terms of our understanding, is very much in the spirit of Erickson's work. The central idea is to do whatever the person needs to have done by letting them do it. The hypnotherapist manages the process and the client does the actual work. The more resourceful a person is, the less the hypnotherapist will have to do. Great hypnotic subjects know what to do when someone invites them to go into trance to resolve an issue. To the degree that all clients are great hypnotic subjects, they will be free to respond in kind. Erickson's work truly embodied the presupposition that every individual has all the resources necessary to change. He was a pioneer of the "individual" and was willing to do whatever it took for each particular individual to change. The use of metaphor completely affirms the individual's abilities, because they choose whatever meaning they take from the metaphors as they go through the change process. A hypnotic interview based upon metaphor is then quite possibly the least intrusive and perhaps the most effective means for change because of its inherent respect of individual choice . . . .

(Suddenly the ceiling lights flicker in the training room.)

Sometimes when clients report a blinding flash of light, it may not just be the ceiling lights. That's when you say, "That was a big one, wasn't it?" Did you know Erickson used to suggest to some of his clients that they would see a blinding flash of light? It was part of his own learning. As a dyslexic child, he could not tell the difference between an M and a 3.[11] He finally realized the M was standing on its legs and the 3 was on its side with its legs sticking out. When he realized the difference between the 3 and the M, he literally saw a blinding flash of light. This happened a few other times as well, where an insight would be accompanied by a blinding flash of light.

Later in his professional career, he used this idea with a woman who was totally bored with her life.[12]

(The ceiling lights of the training room flicker again.)

That's right! Thank you, Dr. Erickson . . . it is your story . . . !

She was having problems with her marriage because her husband wanted to travel and she didn't want to travel. It was a matter of going from Phoenix to Flagstaff—it wasn't like traveling around the world or anything like that. While she was listening intently, *paying attention* to what was immediately important, Erickson told her there would be some point where she would see a blinding flash of color and her life would totally change. By accepting this, her senses were totally heightened, because she was always anticipating seeing this flash of color and having her life change.

She began looking at life with a sense of anticipation and wonder: who knows? *Change could be just around the next corner.* Everywhere she would go she kept looking. Where would she see the flash of color? She looked everywhere . . . . around the world . . . . until finally she did see it. It was a multicolored woodpecker she saw flying across a wooded area. She was thrilled. The change occurred . . . . long before she ever realized it. Only after she had become a seasoned traveler who could *now approach life as a wonderful adventure* did her unconscious mind say, in effect, "We'll let you *have the change now,* let's pick this woodpecker here, it's as good as anything else . . . . it could have easily been . . . ."

Chapter 8
Posthypnotic Suggestion: How To Trans-fer The Learnings

Editor's Notes: This chapter requires minimal preframing as the trainers explain the relevant nuances of posthypnotic suggestion within the chapter itself. The posthypnotic suggestion protocol which they discuss is so effective that the reader may want to review this chapter several times to consciously absorb the information. Seeing the format may explain its utility. It is a series of suggestions which consists of five elements in the following order: trance, new behavior, amnesia, trance, and self-appreciation.

Question to the reader: What might be the purpose of sequencing a posthypnotic suggestion protocol in this way?

In this section, we're going to discuss PostHypnotic Suggestion (PHS), the nature of posthypnotic behavior, and an Ericksonian protocol for PHS. We gleaned the protocol from a number of different sessions which Erickson conducted as well as from his paper on posthypnotic behavior.[1] A posthypnotic suggestion is a suggestion given to someone while they're in trance which is to take effect sometime after they come out of trance. In his book, *Hypnotism,* George Estabrooks had an insightful way of putting it: "There is a rule in hypnotism that everything we get in trance can also be obtained by means of the posthypnotic suggestion. Also, anything that we find in either can be found in autosuggestion; and finally, that everything we obtain in any of the three will be encountered in everyday life."[2]

Erickson's work in the area of posthypnotic suggestion is some of the most important research in the field of Hypnosis. During his years as a researcher at Wayne County General Hospital, he was able to explore the outer limits and the possibilities of posthypnotic suggestion. Until that time, many hypnotists and researchers had made observations about the intriguing qualities of posthypnotic behavior and most agreed that its hallmark was the compulsive nature of its execution.[3] Researchers found that even if the subject knew that a posthypnotic suggestion was given (and even knew what it was), when the time came it would quite likely be carried out.[4] Experimentally, this was the case even when the subject would resist the suggestion. This means that the posthypnotic response is not mediated by higher cortical activity: *when you carry out a posthypnotic suggestion given to you, you act automatically.* Our opinion is that this is true to the extent that the suggestions given are in alignment with the recipient's value system.

Erickson's major contributions focused on his observations and insights into the nature of posthypnotic behavior, particularly those observations about the state the subject was in at the time they performed the behavior. If you're a student of Hypnosis, you'll recognize the significance of his analysis when you read the first few pages of his paper on Posthypnotic Behavior.[5] Erickson was the first to emphasize that, with the arguable exception of research done by Gurney in 1886,[6] **posthypnotic behavior is accompanied by trance** itself. The length of the trance directly relates to the performance of the posthypnotic behavior (the trance will only last as long as the behavior is occurring).

This observation is consistent with what we currently know about state-dependent learning. To produce a behavior, the client has to reaccess the state wherein the behavior was suggested. Erickson conducted experiments where he would interrupt someone who was carrying out a posthypnotic suggestion, and the interruption caused them to stop and go more deeply into trance. This is similar to the pattern interrupt inductions we did earlier. The program (in this case, the posthypnotic suggestion) was interrupted and the person was in a state of temporary suspension until some other cue was given. Dr. Erickson observed that if the person was allowed to complete the behavior (if he removed the interference), the person would immediately resume the posthypnotic behavior, underscoring the compulsive and persistent nature of PHS.

The other feature of posthypnotic behavior which has long fascinated researchers is that posthypnotic behavior is not an integrated part of the situation in which it occurs. In fact, it could be entirely out of the subject's current stream of conscious activity when it happens. Our observation is that the posthypnotic behavior need not in any way be related to the overall context where it is produced. It is related to the context (trance) in which it was generated. The greater the difference between the posthypnotic behavior and where it is executed, the more evident trance formation will be. There may also be some brief confusion and disorientation at the end of the posthypnotic behavior until the subject resumes attention to the immediate context. You'll observe disorientation more typically in demonstrations or in research experiments rather than in the clinical setting.

The reason why disorientation would be less evident after a therapy session is because posthypnotic behavior is directly related to the context where it will be produced. Therefore the behavior will look "normal," automatic, or even conscious, because the behavior is occurring in an appropriate context. That's the intent of getting a well-formed outcome: the behavior is ecological within the context where it was designed to occur. In these cases, trance is still present but less obvious, because the behavior is appropriately integrated and contextualized. If the original hypnotic intervention was done in a light trance, as in most NLP techniques, the depth of trance exhibited in the posthypnotic behavior will be proportionately light. It is important to note that there is no proven relationship between the depth of trance in which the posthypnotic behavior was given and the likelihood that the behavior will be carried out.[7] However, having researched Erickson and many of his notable contemporaries, we have little doubt that they prefer inducing, minimally, a medium level trance and often used amnesia for the trance and the posthypnotic suggestions contained within it. You will see how this is incorporated into our model of Erickson's use of posthypnotic suggestions.

Typically, we prefer giving posthypnotic suggestions toward the end of the trancework. Using our model of the hypnotic interview, posthypnotic suggestions follow whatever changework has been done. Traditionally, the posthypnotic suggestions were the "changework"—they comprised the totality of the intervention. Erickson would often intersperse posthypnotic suggestions throughout the entire hypnotic interview. However, there was often a point toward the end of the trance where he would go through a particular sequence of suggestions. We have found this sequence to be an extremely effective structure with a wide range of clients. We codified it into a protocol that is a useful starting point from which to develop understanding and use of posthypnotic suggestion.

Posthypnotic Suggestion Protocol

1. Trance
2. New behaviors
3. Amnesia
4. Trance
5. Self-appreciation

These are the basic steps. We'll be covering each of these steps in more detail to serve as a trans-later for your conscious mind so you can have a *deeper* understanding of this protocol.

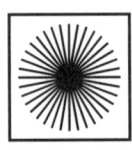

Demonstration of Posthypnotic Suggestion Protocol With Audience

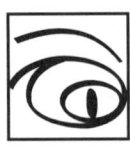

So assuming you were in a trance right now, not necessarily that you are in one (trainers nod heads "Yes") or going into one, but if you were, that way you would understand fully what we're doing here [hear] now what is being said . . . today . . . have you been in a *trance* before? . . . . *Right NOW*. If you have been, then you can continue . . . . . . just sitting there listening intently . . . . If you haven't, you can continue just sitting there, listening intently with your conscious mind, or perhaps you like . . . *letting your mind wander* . . . *your ['re] unconscious* . . . can listen intently to that which is immediately important to it.

The most important thing about anything you've learned here at this seminar isn't that you're going to take these skills and trans-fer them into the real world . . . because what we're much more interested in is your ability to **use hypnosis effectively within yourself** *and to know you have the freedom to go into trance in any way, at any time, that you so choose that's appropriate for you. And you can do that as easily as remembering this word* "**trance**" *. . . said in your mind, in your own way . . . . . .*

. . . . . Or you may have some other way that is your own way of doing it. I don't really know because I only know that you are here primarily to **learn these skills;** *to learn a set of techniques, for example, the hypnotic interview and how to produce hypnotic phenomena . . . or, for example, different types of inductions, so that when you leave here and you see that first client you know is a great hypnotic subject—aren't they all? You'll look across at them and say, "Have you ever been in a trance before? . . . . . Right NOW" . . . . And you'll invite them, as easily as you have here, to go into a trance of their own making so that you both realize that they are great hypnotic subjects. Who knows when you're going to notice that* **these skills have integrated** *and that you're using them easily and in a timely way. Perhaps you'll notice it with the first client you work with or maybe it will be in a couple of weeks from now, after you've really used these skills enough times unconsciously that your conscious mind finally realizes, "Hey, you're using these skills exquisitely." I don't know how you'll realize you're mastering these skills, but I do know that*

you will **use them ethically** and **you will use them effectively to help people change in ways that they want to change.**

But what's far more important than that, really, is to appreciate after your unconscious does it for you ..... In that way, it's so easy to forget. So much so that you've probably forgotten how much you do ...... How many times have you forgotten things? Only to remember exactly what you need to know at precisely the time you needed to know it? After all, you only need to **remember what you know when you need it.** How often do you try to remember your phone number? You don't until it's time to use it. But for that time in between, you just forget it .... **It's easy to forget.** You go to a party, people are introducing themselves to you ..... Have you ever met someone whom you thought was really interesting?..... Remember?.... And you forget about everything else ..... They say, "Hi, I'm so-and-so." At the end of the party, you ask yourself, "What was their name? ..... And what was I talking about earlier?" Sometimes it's just important to let it go and **enjoy yourself.**

After you've had a good meal, you can have the satisfaction of knowing you had a good meal without remembering all the particulars of the meal. You just know it was a satisfying meal, that's it. Let it digest. Let it set. Because sometimes it's just good to let things set. When construction companies build a highway, a new innerstate, they build the foundation and then they lay the concrete and let it set ...... later on even though the concrete could support traffic, they just let it set. Just taking some time to let it set .....

Because trance is like a seed ..... for you to notice the different and varied ways you can experience productive, altered states on your own. Maybe you will learn to do it sitting, maybe you will learn to do it waiting in a line if it's appropriate, I don't know. I only know that you will be able to do it when you want to. Because trance is a learnable skill that you are learning ...... how to go into a trance, easily and comfortably, simply by remembering it ... .. NOW ....!

If you would, just take a few moments to really appreciate not just your unconscious but your conscious mind. Really **appreciate yourself** for the good work that you've done; for who you really are at the deepest level. Appreciate yourself for having invested the time and energy for developing a set of skills that not only can help you but can **help other people.** And what healing effect will that have on other people you've not even met, yet? You'll only know after it happens ...... Until then you can look forward to it. So as you know, all good things must come to an end at some point. Just like watching a good *movie or listening to your favorite song* ...... *You don't necessarily want it to end, but half the fun about coming back out of trance is the anticipation of how much fun it will be experiencing trance the next time.*

So as you notice the tendency to stretch and move about in your seat, that will be the signal from your unconscious mind that it's time to begin to come back outside here .... All the way outside and say, "Hi."

AUDIENCE: Hi!

And that's a very good indication, by the way, that people were in trance. This insignificant posthypnotic suggestion (say "Hi") and the client's willingness to follow through with it can be a gauge for predicting how well or in what way they'll follow through with the other posthypnotic suggestions.

Generally, the deeper the trance, the more literal we become. I remember one time I was a demo subject and I didn't think I was in a deep trance. At that time, I thought I couldn't be in much of a trance if I was hearing everything the trainer was saying to me and if I was aware of my own self-talk. I had already been "in trance" once in the demo, and when he reoriented me the second time he said, "I want you to come back outside and say 'hello,' again." So I came back outside and said, "Hello, again." I thought it was funny that I had repeated "again" and I started laughing. The words just felt like they flew out of my mouth; almost like they were compelled to come out. Immediately my conscious mind rationalized it and said, "Oh well, you know you were just making fun." The conscious mind can make up whatever reason it wants for why it happened. The fact remained that I behaved quite literally and automatically. In an odd way I felt compelled to say it that way, while at the same time I seemed to know what I was doing. That's the nature of posthypnotic behavior and it took me awhile to fully integrate that.

Conceptual Outline of The Posthypnotic Suggestion Protocol

Let's go through the protocol for your conscious mind, so you understand its conceptual design and what effects you can expect from it.

• Trance

When you begin the protocol, start by making suggestions about the subject's improved ability to go into a trance; when, where, how to do it, etc. In NLP terms, you are future pacing self-hypnosis. If you know something about the client's values, it is useful to incorporate them at this point. For example, during the demonstration, we emphasized the idea of having the freedom to go into trance.

• New behaviors

After you've made suggestions oriented around the later development of trance, then begin making direct and indirect suggestions which are relevant to the presenting issue or the purpose of the therapy. Generally it's most useful to frame these in terms of behaviors, even if you're working on other levels, like values, beliefs, and feelings, because behaviors are driven by all of these. Behavior is generally the most observable way of knowing change has taken place. In the demo, we used a number of indirect suggestions: interrogatives such as, "I don't know when, how, where," etc., all of which presuppose that you will learn the skills. The basic idea is to suggest the change by presupposition, while giving choice about specifically how the posthypnotic suggestion will occur. Also in this section are direct suggestions: "You will use the skills ethically and effectively." Interspersed throughout this section (and all of the others) are embedded commands, marked out tonally, which amount to direct suggestions.

• Amnesia

Speaking of amnesia . . .
Think in terms of what we've learned about language so far. Better yet, what were the induction techniques which we did? What are the three induction techniques . . . ?
You'll find that in much of Erickson's clinical work he used amnesia . . . What's the first way to create amnesia? Change the subject—like we just did. Change the subject radically. There are a lot of ways to produce amnesia. First, we'll cover the more process-oriented ones.
Amnesia will often occur spontaneously in conjunction with trance, particularly if you fractionate the client in and out of trance several times.[8] Inducing amnesia in this way is similar to awaking from a dream and "trying" to recall it in the waking state. Many people fail to remember their dreams simply because the state of dreaming is so different and disconnected (via slow wave sleep) from their waking reality. It illustrates the principle of state-dependent learning: you're most likely to remember information when you reaccess the state you were in when you were learning it.
Another similar way to create amnesia is to layer your trancework, create nested loops or use multi-embedded metaphor. Stephen & Carol Lankton's book *The Answer Within*[9] does an outstanding job of delineating multi-em-

bedded metaphor. However, you don't have to be narrating metaphors in order to create this effect. You have been using this construction as early as the third exercise in this training. The primary feature of this construction is symmetry. This means if you start with Pacing Current Experience, then proceed to Revivification and changework. You come back out by reversing the sequence: changework to Revivification and then Pacing Current Experience. You end on the same note with which you had started, i.e. (A-B-C-B-A). Amnesia usually occurs for the information which was in the middle (C), probably because of primacy, recency, and the symmetrical construction of the levels.

If you use open loops—where you begin Metaphor A and don't complete it; begin Metaphor B and don't complete it, give a direct suggestion C, then finish Metaphor B and then Metaphor A—you'll actually create more than amnesia. You will create anticipation when you open the stories and a sense of closure when you finish them. We'll talk more about this when we get to metaphor.

The primary way we're going to create amnesia at this stage of the protocol is through indirect and direct suggestion. The demo we did earlier followed the same approach we used to elicit other hypnotic phenomena. First provide universal examples to activate associations relative to forgetting, pace and lead the client's current experience, and then directly suggest, "It's easy to forget." There were also other language patterns used to create mildly confusing context shifts.

(To audience) Remember the universals and suggestions which were used in the demo?

AUDIENCE: . . . (silence) . . .

You're probably going to have amnesia just because you're doing all these loops! One Ericksonian universal that really worked for me was eating a meal and not having to remember the particulars of the meal. You didn't hear that one? I'll say it again for your conscious minds. *When you have a meal, you can be really satisfied at the end of that meal, but you don't have to review every piece or every nutrient that you've consumed. You just know you've had a wonderful meal.* So the amnesia worked pretty well for some folks. There are lots of good ones like that. Driving down the road and forgetting everything you pass. Making lots of phone calls and forgetting who you called. Forgetting where you put your car keys. Forgetting to take out the trash. Walking into a room and forgetting what you went in the room to get or to do. Pick examples that connect with you—they'll have the greatest impact because you can relate to them and you really believe them.

What is the main direct suggestion for amnesia? "You forget." If you read any of the classic hypnosis literature, you'll notice that they weren't on to the idea of positive internal representations, i.e. saying it the way you want them to think about it. If you read the traditional hypnosis books, you'll notice that one of their main suggestions is, "You can't remember." That can and often does work. It works much better, though, if you direct their attention to where you want it to go: <u>suggesting they'll forget.</u>

Did you hear the part about letting the concrete set?

AUDIENCE: . . . .

That's actually not just for amnesia, but the idea of letting it alone . . . . . when you pave a highway you let the concrete set before you have people drive over it, even though it's solid. It was at the end of the amnesia to let the amnesia set in. An indirect suggestion. Let this alone. Put your attention somewhere else. You don't remember that part?

AUDIENCE: . . . .

• Trance

Once again you're going to suggest trance in much the same way you did at the beginning of the protocol. You're creating a subloop here. It's almost like another trance induction, isn't it? Trance, new behaviors, amnesia, then you complete the subloop with trance. The result is a trance within a trance. You have whatever trance was formed before you got to the posthypnotic suggestion protocol. Now you have another trance (within this protocol), complete with suggestions for amnesia inside of it. This tends to support the development of amnesia. This construction, by the way, conforms with Erickson's experimental findings[10] of how to effectively create posthypnotic behavior accompanied by spontaneous trance. One requisite he believed at that time was amnesia of the initial trance and the posthypnotic suggestions.

Overall, this collapses the new behaviors and amnesia inside of trance. Emphasizing this step via direct suggestion creates the notion that all one is being asked to do is to have the ability to go into trance. However, since the suggestions for the new behaviors are packaged inside of trance instructions, they will be refreshed and reinforced each time the client enters the suggested trance.

• Self-appreciation

The final step to the protocol is self-appreciation. Even if you are not using the entire protocol, this is something worth doing. It encourages alignment between the conscious and the unconscious minds. It encourages self-esteem, providing the opportunity for conscious appreciation of one's abilities, intent, essence, etc., while allowing time for integration of whatever work was done previously. It also ends the experience on a positive note.

Setup For The Exercise

Get together with a new partner this time. We're going to start this exercise the same way we did with the hypnotic interview, except now we're going to include the posthypnotic protocol at the end.

Now let's move beyond "problem" (remedial) and outcome. Do you have anything in your life for which you're preparing? Are you having minor surgery done? Are you making a decision about something? Are you going to be making a speech or a presentation? Are you up for a review at work? Are you beginning any kind of project? Anything which you're preparing for where you want to have more resources available. Any of these would be a good choice for this protocol. What we're looking for is a piece of generative work. In this sense, generative changework starts where you are now and installs processes which will continue to build on themselves as you proceed with the project.

If you decide to work this way, it is still worthwhile to ask if there is anything in the way of installing those processes or achieving the outcome. If you don't get congruency around the outcome, ask "What prevents you?" and design the intervention so it handles it. Use this information to know what theme/reframe to use and what resources need to be accessed. Certainly you can ask your client what they need in the way of resources, if you wish. Then move into the trancework: Conscious-Unconscious Dissociation, utilization of hypnotic phenomena, changework, and then do the new loop in the posthypnotic suggestion protocol.

Is your unconscious mind ready? Okay. Let's take about fifteen minutes each. One, two, three, go.

The Hypnotic Interview And Posthypnotic Suggestion Protocol Exercise

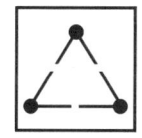

1. Elicitation of the present state and desired state.

2. Conscious-Unconscious Dissociation:
   a. dissociate conscious from unconscious.
   b. anchor problem to conscious mind and solution to unconscious mind.

3. Utilization of hypnotic phenomena:
   a. to deepen trance.
   b. set up direct communication with the unconscious mind.
   c. begin activating resources which support the changework.

4. Changework:
   a. create one major reframe (i.e. separate behavior from intention).
   b. begin unconscious search:
      1. revivify resources.
      2. analogy or metaphor.

5. Posthypnotic suggestion protocol:
   a. trance—the ability to do so when necessary or desired.
   b. new behavior—outcome: both direct and indirect suggestion.
   c. amnesia—universal examples, pacing and leading and direct suggestion.
   d. trance.
   e. self-appreciation.

Do the exercise

Welcome back.

You're welcome, back.

Yes, you are welcome. How did all that go?

They forget, John.

They're still in trance. Everyone just nods their head and has that "trancey" look on their face. Conscious (mind) overload is often another way to induce trance and amnesia.

Speaking of overload . . . overload inductions are fun to do to create amnesia. When I do this with my clients, I start with Conscious-Unconscious Dissociation, which you already know. Then I'll suggest that their unconscious mind can work, for example, on one level to do an unconscious search. While they simultaneously continue this process, at the second level they can begin to revivify resources necessary for their outcome. On the third level, a healing process can occur as their unconscious mind automatically releases negative emotions. I may even suggest a fourth or fifth level, all occurring simultaneously which creates an "overload induction."

This type of induction will definitely create a deeper trance, as well as amnesia, because it buries the conscious mind under so many processes that it can't keep up. Therefore it is particularly useful when doing therapy with people who are very intellectual, and/or who know the NLP skills (i.e. other therapists or trainers), and/or who are smarter than you are! You can do this whenever you think the conscious mind will be too involved in the therapy.

I had a client who really enjoyed the results of this particular technique. He worked at a well-known local institution and his presenting problem was he couldn't get out of bed in the morning to go to work—he was so depressed he would literally stay in bed and not go to work. He was very bright, intellectually gifted, and trained as a therapist. Based upon this, I knew the best therapy would be one in which his conscious mind would not interfere. I saw him four to five times and did overload inductions with him. To preserve the integrity of his work, we did not discuss the session when we were finished. In the fourth session, we did discuss the therapy and his life changes, and by the fifth session, we were complete. Somewhere during the therapy, he resigned at work and started his own private practice. Since then, he has been very successful and has been self-employed now for over three years.

All I did during the therapy was provide suggestions about resolving the issues and improving the quality of his life. I trusted his unconscious mind to figure out exactly how to do it. My job was simply to assist his unconscious mind in removing the blocks which had temporarily prevented him from accessing his internal resources. Fortunately, his rapport with his unconscious mind was strong enough that he could easily align his internal resources and make the necessary changes very quickly. My hunch was that this technique was better for him than a Visual Squash or Time Line Therapy™ because his conscious mind knew those processes so well. I had to use techniques which would totally depotentiate his conscious mind and then his unconscious could do the therapy.

So overload is another way to create amnesia. A handshake induction, such as the Bandler/Grinder version,[11] can also be an overload induction. A double induction—two people talking at the same time—is another example of an overload induction. It creates overload because at first the conscious mind wants to (and thinks it can) listen to both people separately. After a period of time, "trying" to listen to both becomes tiring. At the point of overwhelm, the conscious mind "surrenders" and the person goes more deeply into trance.

AUDIENCE:
How often in a therapy session or how often in general would you use amnesia?

It depends on your client. If you have an intellectual or overly intellectual client, you want to create amnesia as much as possible. If you have someone who is as well trained or better trained than you are, then you may want to use amnesia, because you want to keep the conscious mind out of the way so they're not evaluating the work. You'll want to use amnesia with anyone who is going to get into therapy and think about it a lot.

AUDIENCE:
How long of a session do you need to create amnesia?

Again, it depends on your client. I always start by saying I'm going to ask your conscious or unconscious mind to participate fully here today. That I'm here for you one hundred percent today and whatever turns out will be in your highest and best interest. Then I go into Conscious-Unconscious Dissociation and then into layering a number of different processes on top of one another. Our first session is usually two to three hours and that's plenty of time. With the client I just described, after the initial interview, I saw him for one hour sessions and that worked fine because we did not spend a lot of time discussing content.

AUDIENCE:
At times as the therapist, I was distracted by some of the noise in the room, and I didn't quite know how to handle this with my partner.

There are a lot of ways you can handle it. (Someone's notebook slides off their lap onto the floor.) "Notice old ideas falling away as we speak right now. Notice how easily things can drop off like that?" (The training room windows are open and traffic sounds can be heard in the room.) ". . . . . . . And listen to the cars. Just go ahead and listen to that car driving by . . . . . how it comes and goes . . . . away . . . . just like those problems . . . ."

AUDIENCE:
What about people's voices? . . . Loud voices . . . ?

"Perhaps you haven't considered listening to the people's voices . . . that were in the background because that way it would be so much easier for trance to occur. Your conscious mind may already be distracting itself while it engages in a peripheral conversation, so that I can *speak directly to your unconscious.*" Or, if you were the hypnotherapist, you could say, "Go ahead and listen to those other people . . . . . because it's fun to listen in on different conversations and you can get a little bit from this person . . . . or a little bit from that person . . . and maybe none of it will make any sense to you at all consciously . . . . but it can be enjoyable and make you curious about what's being said . . . . . because I want to talk to your unconscious . . . . ."

When you read most Hypnosis books, the first step to inducing trance is usually to "fixate attention." Unfortunately, people can at times engage in what we refer to in NLP as "eating the menu." They mistake the "map for the territory" and rotely expect their clients to stare at a point on the wall, as if fixation of attention is only visually staring at a point. Then when a person doesn't want to stare at a point on a wall, the hypnotherapist thinks the client is refractory. In fact, if you have a sound that you know is intrusive, it's perfect because you don't have to ask them to focus on a point on the wall. You have something that is already drawing or fixating their attention and you just have them use that.

When a person comes in with pain, it's going to be much easier to start the induction by having them temporarily focus on the pain than it is trying to get them to relax. That's probably not where their conscious awareness is. It might be where you want to take them, but if you're going to pace them, you've got to start where they are. If they're aware of this chronic pain, that's probably where you're going to want to start and that's where you have them fixate their attention. Wherever they want to fixate their attention is all right with you. Sometimes it is the "distractions" that can be the attractions. You can use "distractions" similarly to trigger posthypnotic suggestions, especially if they're predictable or repetitive.

In my previous office, I had an answering machine. It was on the other side of the room, but it was very loud and obvious when it would go on and off. Finally, I accepted that it could happen at any time when I was doing hypnosis. When it went off during an induction with a person, I would say, ". . . And your attention can wander to your foot, to your right hand, to your left hand".... and then it would go BOOOOOP very loudly and then make these loud clicking sounds. "...... And continue wandering to the sound of the answering machine. . . . ." Later on I would say, *"I wonder what new insights or pleasant associations will be triggered the next time you hear the answering machine click on* . . . . . or maybe you'll just smile at this preposterous notion and enjoyably go deeper . . . ." I had one woman who left one day and was disappointed because we didn't get any more calls! I often wish I would have left her a message a few days later on her machine which would have begun, *"And that was not a posthypnotic suggestion . . . . .!"* Certainly not a posthypnotic suggestion to *trans-fer the learnings, now!*

Chapter 9

Constructing Stories: What Is A Metaphor, Anyway?

"... Metaphor is not just pretty poetry ..."
Gregory Bateson, 1987[1]

Editor's Notes: This chapter details how to create, develop, and deliver metaphors. The Trainers emphasize that creating the context in which the metaphor will be told is as important as what metaphor is told. The reader will note an exercise on "the structure of bushy-brained," which is a phrase used by some in the NLP community to denote a special type of creativity. The Master Woodcutter metaphor sequence models a structure Erickson used, which the Trainers refer to as the Metaphorical Interview in Chapter Ten.

Question to the reader: Why is metaphor an effective means for change? How many loops remain open at the end of the chapter?

There are many of us who have studied Dr. Erickson's work and are not "first generation Ericksonians." In other words, we didn't have direct contact with him while he was living. His work became so legendary that we somehow concluded that creating metaphor meant creating a grand tapestry of seamless wisdom, which perhaps only someone like Milton Erickson could have developed. We thought that those of us with common intelligence could create such metaphors only after endless hours of persistent composition.

One of the things we like to ask people to do at Trainers' Training is to develop five short metaphors which would be suitable for the context of an NLP training. People get very concerned and rush out to their favorite bookstores, thinking, "I've got to go out and buy some new books and find some metaphors!" (When we went though Trainer's Training, we did the same thing.) It took us a long time to realize that often the best ones are staring you in the face. You're living them every minute of your life. Many times they're slices of life to which we can all relate. Metaphors are everywhere: in fact, considering "What isn't a metaphor?" is probably a more difficult proposition. For those of us who struggled with this it seems much like the case of the fish asking, "Where's the water?"

By the way, metaphors aren't just the kind that last thirty to forty-five minutes. More often, they're slices of life which last thirty seconds, a minute and a half, two minutes, or five minutes. For the most part, weaving together a number of short stories will generally be more effective because people can relate to those. It requires less investment on their part to listen to a series of metaphors than to listen to one long story.

We feel that you'll be much more effective when you view metaphors in this way. Any slice of life can be a metaphor. At some point, you will hear a great story or maybe it will just happen when you're working with a client. That's fun because something will come out of your mouth and you'll think to yourself, "This is going to be a great metaphor. I'm going to use this." Other times, it might be a very brief, "no big deal" type of incident, which you look at from a number of different perspectives—kind of like the *Seinfeld* show, if you've ever seen that on television.

You now have roughly fifteen to twenty universal experiences from the examples which you developed in the hypnotic phenomena section. Those are all metaphors or potential metaphors. They're little bullet metaphors, which you could expand upon if you wanted. As an example, we can talk about time distortion. Think of a time when you were on a long trip, driving sixty mph on the highway for quite awhile. Suddenly you get off onto an exit ramp where the speed limit is thirty-five mph, and what does your sensation of movement feel like? That's right—it feels so much slower that it seems that you have much more time to think and react. That's a brief metaphor to which you could add some interesting details about where you were going, or who you were going to see, and so on. Then you can move on to another short story about a time when your watch stopped and what that experience was like. You could have four or five (or more) slices of life sequenced together, all with the common theme of time distortion. This is an effective way to have people pay attention to what is immediately important.

We're going to approach metaphor a bit differently from the standard texts. We're not going to give you a heavily detailed way to construct metaphors. Instead, we'll give you what we think are some important points and guidelines about metaphors and leave the rest up to your creativity and sensory acuity—the Ericksonian approach to teaching metaphor!

Metaphor construction and presentation are skills which are not generally emphasized, even in psychotherapy. If you want to find strategies for constructing and presenting metaphors, study oral traditions like storytelling. Before written literacy, all important information was transmitted orally. The work of storytellers was always a balance between remembrance and improvisation, and knowing how to present information in a way so that it could be retained. Rather that just being focused on content, oral poets relied on such aspects as rhythm, repetition, surprising twists, the playing of opposites against each other, mnemonics, and tying the story to what was important and familiar to the listener. They understood that these elements made it easy for the listener to remember the story. In many traditions, the oral poets wouldn't bother with verbatim memorization because many times there wasn't an original written text to begin with! Experts in oral tradition claim that with each repetition, only one-half to two-thirds of a story is reproduced.[2,3] This is why people would often report discrepancies in Erickson's account of the cases which he used for teaching or healing stories. The context determines how the story is told. The speaker calibrates to the client or the audience and observes their cues. Then he or she utilizes the audience's responses and tailors the details of the metaphor to that particular audience.

In Ong's book, *Interfaces of the Word: Studies in the Evolution of Consciousness and Culture*,[4] he mentions that some of his students accompanied some well-known storytellers for a certain period of time. They found the same story could vary from ten minutes to an hour and a half, depending on the audience's response. One student said, "You always knew ahead of time what he was going to say, but you never knew how he would say it or how long it would take."[5] This is what makes using therapeutic metaphors so much fun. Each time becomes a one-time performance—the next retelling will always be different from the last. The stories you tell will grow as you grow, and that is what will make them effective. Many times it will be this spirit in the telling which will have the most profound impact on your client.

A Strategy For Brewing The Spirit of Your Story

1. Find a story, incident, or slice of life which had an impact on you.
2. Read it over or go over it once mentally.
3. Let it settle in—at least overnight.
4. Recall it again and notice:
   a. what are the major themes?
   b. what other associations (other incidents, stories, etc.) do they stimulate in you?
5. Let it settle in, again, overnight.
6. Tell the story. Realize it's a "once-only" performance. The next time you tell it, it will be different.

This method is useful when you've got some time for incubation to further refine your stories. We're reminded of some of the Hawaiian healers we studied. It was not unusual for them to see the client initially to determine the problem and then ask them to return at another time for the actual intervention. The practitioner would meditate or dream on the client's case and see them in the next day or so. The Hawaiians understood the utility of letting the spirit brew, having the client wait for the healing set the stage, and thereby creating the context for the intervention to be a meaningful experience.

Setting The Stage:
How Do You Spell "Meaning"? . . . . C O N T E X T

Unfortunately, most people spend more time on the content of the metaphor, when the most critical element is the context which is created when the content is related. If you've read any books on metaphor construction, you may remember that they all mention the importance of isomorphism.[6] What this means is that the metaphors chosen need to have "like form" or structural correspondence to the client's situation. For example, if growing up was an issue for a child, then a like structure would be the process of trees growing and maturing. An isomorphic structure insures the metaphor will have meaning for the client and provides a framework for a new response.

It's easy to take this to mean that the content of the metaphor needs to have similarities with the client's situation. While this is true, be aware that the context which you create before you deliver the story, as well as how you deliver the metaphor, will be equally critical in creating meaning and the framework for a new response. The global context involves the overall setting in which you present the metaphor, as well as any preframing you may do. "How" you deliver the metaphor is contingent upon nonverbals, such as smiling, tone of voice, use of silence, etc. Remember, all meaning is context dependent.[7] In fact, before we go any further, let's consider how and why metaphors work.

I had a client whose presenting issue was her ideal weight. Over a period of sessions, she had done very well at achieving and maintaining her ideal weight, and it was no longer the emphasis of therapy. She was an administrator for a health-care institution and was quite motivated and eager to do what was asked of her. She was very creative but not in a system which was willing to support her creativity. She was feeling overwhelmed by the conflict between all the possible changes which could be made and a system which she perceived as inflexible. Her presenting issue for this session was "overwhelm."

Around the time she came in with that issue, I listened to a tape by Steve Lankton.[8] On that tape, Steve said he wondered if Dr. Erickson really knew what he expected his clients to do ahead of time when he assigned tasks or ordeals. Did he really have a clue? Steve started to consider that sometimes Erickson didn't but was so good at utilization that, no matter how the client responded to the ordeal, he would find some way to make it work. Lankton then suggested that in certain cases it may be appropriate for one to pick something which is totally (or seemingly) unrelated to the therapy and ask the client to do it and find out what happens—as long as it's ethical and safe. I had just heard this and, sitting with my client, I thought, *"This is an opportunity to learn something."*

So here's my client with the overwhelm. She was a model client who would listen to NLP tapes and was familiar with a number of the patterns we were using in the therapy. I remember at one point in the therapy she smiled and said, "Great double bind."

We began the session by just talking about her overwhelm. We talked and she analyzed and considered everything which was going on until we had about five minutes left in the session. I knew I could still give her an ordeal and we could end the session on that note. I told her, "When you get home, I want you to go find a new box of Kleenex. Take a bunch of Kleenex and roll them up into a ball; just crumple them into a ball. Do you have a table in your kitchen?" She said, "Yes." "Before you go to bed tonight, I want you to put it on the kitchen table because you want to get rid of all this (the overwhelm), right?" She said. "Yes." I continued, "Put the ball of Kleenex in the middle of your kitchen table and then go to bed. Once you wake up the next morning, before you leave the house, I want you to take that same ball of Kleenex, find a drawer in the kitchen, put it in the drawer, close the drawer, and leave it in there all day until it's time to go to bed; at which time, I want you to open the drawer back up, take the Kleenex back out and put it out on the table so it stays out all night." The other thing I told her (for her conscious mind) was, "I want you to consider what relationship this has to your therapy." Then she left.

My thought process behind assigning her this task was similar to what Steve Lankton had recommended. I just picked something I thought was as far removed from what she was saying as I could imagine. The idea of the Kleenex was just something that flew into my head and I thought, "Okay, what the heck, let's do it."

She came back two weeks later, and I thought she looked like she was doing pretty well. When assigning ordeals, you have to be very careful what you ask the client so that you don't undermine any presuppositions of the work. As she walked into my office, I asked her how things were going and her verbatim reply was, "Things have really settled down." "Really?" I said with some surprise and curiosity.

She replied, "Yeah, things have really settled down." I said, "That's interesting. How did you do it?" We talked for a little while and she said, "You know that thing you had me do? I said, "What are you talking about?" She said, "The Kleenex thing." I said, "Yes." She said, "Well, I went home, and did exactly what you said. I put it out on the table and the next morning I put it in the drawer. When I came home that night, I took it out and put it on the kitchen table. The next day (maybe it was the second, third, or fourth day), I woke up, got ready for work, and I had a meeting I had to get to. I got in my car and I drove off and halfway to work I realized I had forgotten to put the Kleenex in the drawer. So I turned around, went back home and put it in the drawer, and then I went back to work."

I said, "Mm, hmmm...." Then I asked, "What happened next?" (Author's note: I'm not sure if she said this happened the next day or if it was a couple of days later.) She answered, "Once again I got up and had to speed off to work, and I realized I had forgotten it again. I forgot to do it, again! At that moment she said, "___ it, I'm not doing that anymore!" With that she drove right to work... and that was it. No more overwhelm.

Most clients come to you because they are where they are and they want to be somewhere else in their lives. They are at point A and want to get to point B. They are holding these two things in mind—where they are and where they want to be. Together, these create a context. To the extent that you have rapport with them (which further defines context) and they are invested in the process of changing, anything which you introduce relative to those two things will stimulate their unconscious mind to ask, "How does this relate to what we're doing?" That's why what you pick as a metaphor may not be as important as the context you create before you tell it and while you're telling it.

The "Kleenex task" was a "living metaphor" where she had to physically participate in the metaphor; yet it *was* a metaphor. I didn't know what it meant to her, but it apparently meant enough that she had a breakthrough. I didn't ask her about the specific meaning which it had for her. My guess is it was another example of doing something someone asked her to do which she thought she had to do perfectly. This time she realized there were things which were important and there were things she could let go of which weren't important (the task and the overwhelm). That's my mind read on how she interpreted the task, but really that's academic. If I would have tried to construct a metaphor with that moral, I don't know if I could have done it as well as she did. As long as you have rapport and have suggested to your client (often the context itself will do this) that the story you're about to tell has relevance for their situation, you can them find their own meaning in their own way.

Let's take a closer look at what created the proper context. Rapport was very important. Using this intervention wasn't something I would have or could have done right off the bat. I had seen her for several hours previous to the ordeal, and she had invested herself in the process and had a reason not to leave the "field." These conditions are necessary not only in ordeal therapy but also in double binds, metaphorical interventions, and probably for therapy in general.

Ordeals and metaphors are also very useful if you've reached an impasse in therapy. An impasse signals that the relationship has found its growing edge. So whatever you do, as long as you *do something* and *do it with sincerity* from a dynamic point of view, it will be therapeutic (and metaphorical in that sense). You calibrate to your client and, based on who you are and who they are, *let your unconscious come out with the answer. Trust it and go with it and learn something.*

The main criteria we hold in our minds for choosing "living metaphors" or ordeals are: Is it ethical? Is the physical task itself something that is positive, helpful, or at least benign? If it is, then I'm willing to do it. You don't do ordeals just to do ordeals, however. In many cases, you can create a "win-win" situation when you've reached an impasse if you're willing to do something differently. An important requirement is that it doesn't have to have an obvious or direct relationship to the therapeutic issue.

The point here isn't so much about ordeals and how to do them, but rather that the ordeal served as a metaphor. Her *unconscious mind* was willing to put whatever meaning it needed into what was offered: *get what meaning you need to get out of it* and get to the next point. That's all a metaphor is.

This is what we enjoy so much about working this way. Metaphor and other forms of ambiguity provide the forum for the listener's unconscious mind to participate fully or not; to assign meaning based upon their experiential understandings; and to reorganize these understandings to create a new schema for perceiving the world.

Metaphor affirms a person's resourcefulness and creativity and increases the likelihood that the learnings will be remembered. Unconscious presentation of information for problem-solving generates a greater mobilization of resources than simple presentation of information at the conscious level.[9] Analogical structures, in general, are more effective in integrating relevant information from short-term to long-term memory (i.e. if we told a story about this study, you'd remember this principle better).[10]

The Optimal State For Doing Metaphors: "Bushy-brained"

Bushy-brained is a useful state and you won't find it on a map. It's the ability to look at something differently, perhaps even slightly askew. The rest of the world calls it "creativity" because they think something like creativity doesn't grow on trees, shrubs, or bushes (hence "bushy"-brained!) Personally, we think it does, and quantum physicists and Vedic scientists would probably agree.

Let's do an exercise to get warmed up for constructing metaphors. Creativity (bushy-brainedness) is correlated with the ability to simultaneously hold in thought two or more opposite or dissimilar concepts.[11] This exercise is based upon that premise. Being in this kind of state makes therapy fun and will definitely loosen up your thinking. It gives insight into how a problem and solution can relate to one another. The skills inherent in this exercise—chunking up to higher logical levels and then chunking laterally—have been cited as universally effective ways to think creatively. Edward DeBono coined the term "lateral thinking" for this process.[12]

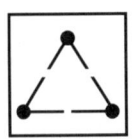

Bushy-brained Exercise

We'll have you form groups of three. This is an uptime exercise although it will produce an interesting effect in your head. At the count of three, two of the people will each say a noun, a thing, anything, it doesn't matter what it is. It can be specific or abstract. We'll do it for you quickly:

1-2-3 . . . . shoe
1-2-3 . . . philosophy

So we've got "shoe" and "philosophy." The third person in the group will consider what the words have in common. How are shoe and philosophy alike—what do they have in common?

AUDIENCE: They're a foundation of activities . . . or . . . you have to dig into it . . . or . . . they can both be stretched.

It looks like you've got it. That's the exercise. It's a really good way to tune your brain and it will put you in an upstate so when you walk out of here you'll feel wide awake. Everybody got that? Take five to ten minutes.

Do the exercise

Discussion

How was that? Fun? Sort of loosens up the stuff in there, doesn't it? What were some of your responses?

"Cemetery" and "eyes." Commonality: pupils. Irises growing among the pupils.
"Purple shoes" and "a can." You can-can; you can dance in purple shoes.
"Turnips" and "speakers." So you can "turn-ip" the volume of your speakers. On that note, let's move on to the next step!

How To Deliver The Metaphor

We will go into more detail about sequencing and utilizing metaphors in a later section. At this point, let's cover some of the basic elements in delivering metaphors. First, everything that you've learned about indirect hypnotic methods applies. One of the most powerful determinants of the context is what you do nonverbally, with your physiology and your voice. As you begin, match and mirror the client and then begin to model the physiology of the state which corresponds with the metaphor or the part of the metaphor you're telling. Calibrate to your client and notice how they react, both consciously and unconsciously, to what is being said. This will help you know how long to stay on one part versus another. If they get the point right away, there's no reason for you to keep going on about the same point unless your objective is to bore them into trance, so to speak. This is why we talked earlier about the importance of knowing the general themes and associations to the metaphor. You'll fill in the details as you go. One other point may seem obvious. You ought to know, at least generally, how the story ends, especially if it has a punch line!

Using Multi-Embedded Metaphor

It's not the scope of this training to teach you a specific protocol for multi-embedded metaphors. The definitive work on that topic has already been done by Stephen and Carol Lankton. We highly recommend that you read *The Answer Within*[13] if you want to study this in detail.

We'd like to suggest to you that this entire training has been done in multi-embedded metaphors, also known as nested loops. If you pick the structure of any of the early exercises, you will find the same parallel layering effect, so you can create this effect without having to use metaphors. The rule of thumb is that the steps you lead the client through on the way into the induction are reversed when you begin to reorient them. For example, if you induce trance by doing metaphor A, then metaphor B, then metaphor C, you come back out continuing with metaphor C, then metaphor B and end with metaphor A. In this construction, you have different themes and information packaged at different levels. Ong said, "The epic is built like a Chinese puzzle—boxes within boxes."[14] As we discussed earlier, this parallel layering effect usually produces amnesia, particularly for the segments in the middle. In our A-B-C-B-A construction, example C would likely become the most unconscious; followed by B; with A usually being what is likely to be remembered because of primacy and recency.[15]

A slight variation on the concept of parallel layering and multi-embedded metaphor is the open loop. This is when you begin a story and, at the chosen point, break off into another metaphor without finishing the first one. This has interesting effects on the listener. To the extent that you do this a number of times, and your transitions are smooth, you will induce trance via overload as the conscious and unconscious minds listen for the conclusion of the stories. Some believe this may prevent premature closure on a subject.

If you use open loops with new clients or new audiences, it is generally a good idea to use smooth transitions or else you might seem, to your audience, to be scattered or on drugs! You could also preframe that at times you will be starting some stories and perhaps not finishing them. They are a useful convention and can produce curiosity and "cliff-hanger"-like drama. We like open loops and use them a lot. Let's see: how many loops do we have open right now? . . . Is that another open loop?

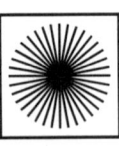

Demonstration of Multi-Embedded Metaphor With Audience

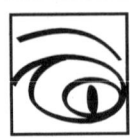

I'm not sure if these stories were ever told **inside** the garage, but my understanding is that up in the northwestern part of the United States at some time, I'm not sure if it's this time, there lived a man who was known as the Master Woodcutter. He truly was a master at his craft, and students from all around would go to meet the master and to hear him tell of his experiences. That's how he taught his students until they were ready to become masters themselves.

There was one enterprising student, new to the field, who decided to go visit the Master Woodcutter. He had to drive some distance to get there. Eventually he travelled up this long road which took him up to the top of a hill. It was heavily wooded, just as you would imagine in the Pacific Northwest where there are tall evergreens, tall trees, very green.

The student was told, "You'll know you've arrived when you see this old chap sitting there on his front porch in a rocking chair . . . . . ." Looking down on a small village below . . . . . . you could see fields down below as well as the trees behind. And there was the Master Woodcutter, already sitting with a number of students who seemed to be focused intently on what was being said.

Constructing Stories: What Is A Metaphor, Anyway?

After sitting for awhile, thoughts and questions began to stream through the student's mind: what is he doing? He's not teaching anything, he's just telling stories. How will I ever learn anything this way? Finally the student felt he had to ask a question. It was something that had been bugging him and he needed clarification. Just as he began to ask, the Master Woodcutter said, *"Just **stop**, and just **listen** to a couple of things first and perhaps you'll discover that you already have the answers to some of the questions you had. There are two things you need to be able to do and understand to become a Master Woodcutter."* The student sat there waiting and the Master Woodcutter paused appropriately . . . . then said, "The <u>first</u> thing is you have to be willing to *learn something. You have to be able to learn from anything to become a Master* Woodcutter." He looked at the student and said, "You do want to become a master, do you not?" . . . . (Trainer calibrates to audience) . . . . Some just sat there, some nodded their heads . . . .

"To become a Master Woodcutter you have to be *willing to learn from anything.* For example (Trainer slowly points out the window) . . . . just look over there . . . ." (waits for audience to look) . . . . He said, "Look at those hedges way down over the hill there. See those hedges down there? Those shrubs? They need to be trimmed." The students thought, "What the hell is he talking about?" (pacing students' mild confusion) "Just go ahead and see those hedges there, shrubs that need to be trimmed. They belong to a friend of mine who's name is Mabel. A few years ago, Mabel invited me down to her house and she told me there were some *new developments* she wanted to tell me about. So I traveled *all the way down* and knocked on her front door. Looked at the hedges and thought, 'Need some pruning.' No one answered the door at first. Knocked again. No answer . . . . everything was quiet in there."

Being a Master Woodcutter, being intuitive and a friend of Mabel, he decided to let himself *go inside* Mabel's house, and there was Mabel sitting in a chair staring off into the distance through this big window. And off in front of her were these fields . . . . . she was just sitting . . . . *looking straight ahead. Quietly.* And he walked up to her and asked, "How are you, Mabel?" She said, "Oh, I'm glad you're here. There are some new developments, some changes . . . . but before I tell you what they are . . . . just stop for a moment and look, just look at the wheat fields out there. Now they're getting ready to harvest that wheat out there; it's soon harvest time. You can feel it in the air." She looked out there and asked, "Can you see the kids out there? You may not see them at first . . . . . . got their coats on . . . *nice and warm* . . . . winter's on it's way . . . . ."

". . . . I remember all the winters that those kids were out there, playing in the snow, making snowballs, making snowmen . . . . just being kids . . . . . having fun . . . . and in the spring, we'd all go out and plant seeds together

. . . . and the summer . . . . . watching the crops grow and enjoying the warm, sunny days . . . . . and then it's fall . . . . time to harvest . . . . . ."
 She had a tone to her voice . . . . full of emotion . . . . The Woodcutter started wondering where she was going with all of this.
 She looked at him and asked, "When's the last time we just sat and reminisced? Remember all those good times we had over there behind the stove—the big wood stove that was really the heart of this house—where everybody would get together? I remember when the kids would come in and bring the wood in the winter and it would *get nice and warm inside* . . . . . . and the dining room table, look at that dining room table and all the scratches." She said, "I could tell you a story about how each one of the scratches got on that table. I remember all the dinners we had there, all the holiday dinners, people that were gathered, the turkey or the ham, mashed potatoes, smells that came in."
 Then they walked over through the kitchen. "Let me take you back outside for just a moment." She opened the door: the old screen door went, "rrrrrrrr," squeaking loudly. She said, "I've got to do something about that squeaky door . . . . . . but I guess everyone has a squeaky door . . . . " She went outside and said, *"Just look at the beauty that's around us. Really look at it."*
 "Look at those trees out there. See those big giant evergreens out in front of you? Twenty for a nickel. That's back in the old days when you used to be able to buy twenty of those little trees for a nickel. Look how much they've grown now. But there's really only nineteen, if you count them, because one died . . . . . had to make room for the others. Look at that compost pile we've got going there now. Now a lot of the city folks, they don't appreciate how long it takes to get a good compost pile going and how useful it can really be."
 "Let's go back inside." So she took the Master Woodcutter back inside, opened the screen door. The screen door squeaked. "Got to do something about that screen door one of these days. It's been like that for so long."
 As they walked back inside the house, she said, "Now I want to tell you about this new development." The Master Woodcutter asked, "What is it?" By now, he thought it was about time she told him. She continued, "I'm moving on. *It's time for a change.*" The Master Woodcutter asked, "Do you want some help in moving on?" as he waited for a nod.
 He continued, "You do have an attic up there, don't you? I bet you haven't cleaned it out yet, have you? Maybe not for a long time. Here's a suggestion: "Think this over first before you do it. Go up there to the attic and look at all the stuff you've got up there . . . . all those memories . . . . . . all those things you thought you should hold on to or maybe you didn't know what to do with . . . . I want you to make three piles. The first pile ought to be the biggest pile. Just pile it up. That's *all the stuff that you don't need anymore.* Put that in the trash and let the trash man take it away. *Just get rid of it.* Trash removal is

so much more efficient these days. There's always recycling, too. *Put it all out before you go to bed tonight and when you wake up **tomorrow, it's gone.***
"The second pile can actually be a little bit smaller. *The second pile will be all the things that are no longer of use to you that you'd like to give to someone else who could make good use of them*—you know, a collection for Goodwill. It's always appreciated. *Good will come by . . . . just set up a time . . . . . and you can **write it off**.* Make sure you get a receipt.

"And the third pile is the smallest pile . . . . . . *just the things you are going to take with you . . . . . . so you're comfortable as you move* on . . . . it's easier when you travel lightly . . . . if you forget anything, most *stores are open* seven days a week and other *stores are open all night . . . . . **just go inside and get what you need when you need it.***"

So Mabel thought about it for awhile and gave him a look that she was ready . . . . Up the steps she went to get into the attic . . . . and she stepped inside and the door closed . . . .

Every now and then, it was evident that there was a lot of quiet activity going on . . . things being moved . . . shifted around . . . ready to go . . . . . The woodcutter just waited . . . . . . his mind wandering from one subject to the next . . . waiting for Mabel to finish the job . . . waiting for the attic door to open . . . . .

Before he knew it . . . . he really wasn't sure how much time had gone by . . . . . . the door opened . . . . and Mabel walked back down the steps. "All done?" he asked. "All done."

"Then there's one other thing you need to do. **Say 'Good-bye.'** There are different ways to say good-bye. Everybody has their own way. Some people just wave. Some say it with tears. Some smile and blow a kiss. Some say 'Adios.' Some say, 'Hasta la vista.' Some say, 'Auf Wiedersehen.' In Hawaii they say, 'Aloha,' which is also a way to say 'Hello.'

"First, look at the piles of stuff and say 'Good-bye.' And look out at the wheat fields and say 'Good-bye.' Go ahead and say 'Good-bye' to the children playing out there, planting seeds in the spring, say 'Good-bye'. . . . . . . and . . . . 'Good-bye' to the summers . . . . When you turn around, you look there, see the hearth, and all the wood . . . . say 'Good-bye'. . . . say 'Good-bye' to the dining room table and all the scratches and all the holidays . . . . and as we go outside, rrrrrr (the squeaky door) say 'Good-bye' to the trees, to the nineteen that lived and the one that died, say 'Good-bye' . . . . say 'Good-bye' to the old compost heap . . . say 'Good-bye'. And as they opened the door, it squeaked, rrrr rrr . . . . Say 'Good-bye' to that squeaky door you never bothered to get to. Say 'Good-bye' to that, too."

The Woodcutter knew she was ready . . . . . a look of resolve came over her face. The time had come . . . . . ***time to move on*** . . . . . . they gave each other a hug and said, "Good-bye."

A year or so went by, and once again Mabel came to visit him. They were driving down there in the valley and they went through the village where Mabel used to live. As they passed her house, she pointed at the hedges and said, "<u>**Their**</u> hedges need trimming. They had better tend to <u>their</u> hedges."

It was at that point the Master Woodcutter knew that she had moved on because it was "<u>their</u>" hedges which needed trimming. They were no longer hers because she had said, "Good-bye."

The student was just sitting there, letting all those things go through his mind . . . .

The Master Woodcutter said, "Before we stop for now, look at all those trees . . . . . . See all these big trees out here? . . . . . . Reminds me of a Native American Nation which lives in Northern California. They really understand trees. And if you really want to become a Master Woodcutter, you should know what they know. They have a practice that might seem strange to an outsider. They like to systematically set forest fires. To most people that seems like a bizarre thing to do. But they understand something we don't understand: they *understand nothing really dies and that* **change is natural**. They knew that from the trees, watching from season to season, the endless cycle of transformation. They knew it from watching the day give way to night and the night give way to day . . . an endless cycle of transformation.

"They would look at a forest or woods or a small grove of trees and were able to make important distinctions. They *learned the difference between healthy growth and unhealthy growth* just by looking, by feeling and by listening. They were able to understand the relationship between the forest and themselves. They were able to understand that they were the caretakers of the forest, but they were not the owners of it. After all it had a mind of it's own . . . . . its nature . . . .

"After *care fully* surveying the exterior of the forest, they would *go deep into the interior* . . . . and would decide what is healthy growth and what is unhealthy growth . . . . finding the areas where most of the unhealthy growth proliferated . . . . having identified the unhealthy growth, they would even ask the trees, 'Is it okay for you to be transformed?' and wait for a sign that permission was granted . . . .

"They would mark out certain boundaries or buffers to contain the unhealthy growth by using a stream, or building a wall. Sometimes they would even make a backfire so the fire would only burn in the area needing transformation and leave the surrounding areas untouched.

"Then they would start a small fire within the un*healthy growth and let nature take its course. Nothing ever dies. It gets transformed* . . . . **change is natural.**

"And as the fire burned . . . . from a *safe* distance they would watch the flames of transformation . . . . . . listening to the crackling . . . and feeling the *warmth . . . . inside.* They knew that nothing really dies, it just gets transformed . . . . change is natural . . . . the life of the burning trees contained in the ash would once again return to the soil where it had started and where it would once again become the basis of new life, new growth generations to come . . . . *while the fire burned, the vision of the future would be the only focus . . . . . . and life goes on."*

And with that the Master Woodcutter sat quietly and waited for the students to fully absorb what was said. Finally one of the students broke the reverie and said, "Well, this is great, I'm really glad you told me all of this but what is the <u>second</u> thing I need to know to be a Master . . . . Woodcutter?"

After you've completed this training in trance, remember that Dr. Erickson did all of his work inside the garage. But you don't have to have a garage to do great work with your clients—both of you can **go inside** anywhere and get the same results.

And when you're working with folks, you're going to see them go through a lot of different changes and you may, too. Be willing to **learn from anything** . . . . When you find those things you no longer need or you want to give away, all that you have to do is **say "Good-bye"**. . . . . **Nothing really dies. It's just transformed, the change is natural.**

Analysis of Metaphor Sequence

There are several points we'd like to make while your unconscious mind continues to process this information. Because perhaps you didn't know that your unconscious mind continues to search for information at a rate of thirty items per second even after your conscious mind thinks it knows the answer.[16]

As we noted earlier, metaphor encourages experiential participation rather than restricted intellectual understanding. It simultaneously engages the intellect through curiosity, suspense, drama, and even mild confusion as it questions, "What does this really have to do with me? Is he really talking to me or what?" What is valuable is that the conscious mind wonders about the content, while the unconscious mind participates on another level in whichever way is meaningful to it. As the transformational linguists have said, the deep structure for any pronoun is always "I." To make meaning, we have to try it on. Therefore some of the ways to use metaphors are:

1. Perceptual change—through the absorption in the story, the listener's state is altered and trance is induced.
2. Affective change—evoking different emotional states through the emotional content of the story.

3. Behavioral change—suggesting a series of steps, i.e., a strategy, leading to a specific outcome. The strategy is rehearsed through the actions of the characters.
4. Cognitive change—offering different points of view, i.e., reframing and installation of empowering beliefs and values.

As in other indirect methods, you may first want to momentarily divert conscious attention after ending the metaphors. Second (and some would say that this is a cardinal rule when using metaphors), do not explain what they mean to the client after you're finished. It may be a temptation, because you might think the message is quite powerful and relates to your client's situation. Unfortunately, if you decipher it for them, you've defeated the entire purpose for using metaphor as a therapeutic intervention in the first place. How much fun was it when family members told what you were going to get for Christmas just before *you're ready to open the present?* Wouldn't it have been better if they let you open it yourself? With your clients, the only present you need to open is your present. Let them open theirs. Ambiguity is a wonderful thing.

Since we also told you the Master Woodcutter metaphors for teaching purposes, let's look at the sequence. Let's just hit the high points because there is a fair amount happening on a number of levels. There were three main metaphors with a number of subloops in each of them. The sequence opened with the student and the Master Woodcutter. The purpose was, of course, to match the student-teacher relationship with the Master Woodcutter offering two pieces of advice on how to become a Master Woodcutter. The first answer was provided immediately, and you may or may not have noticed that the second has not been revealed yet (so that loop is still open). Many of the details in the metaphor change each time I do it, because I plug in what I observe going on in the room. How the student arrives and how the conversation goes changes each time. All I know is that I'm going to introduce the student and the Master Woodcutter and open the loops on the two things you need to know to become a Master Woodcutter. This is an example of a pacing metaphor, as well as a teaching metaphor to communicate certain attitudes or beliefs about learning.

I've utilized this metaphor alone and within relationship contexts other than the teacher-student. It's probably important to note here that I had been using all three of these metaphors separately for some time. Then one time I did them in the above sequence and liked the results, so I expanded on them a bit further.

The second metaphor, Mabel saying "Good-bye," is an adaptation of a story Erickson told of his mother, Martha, that has also been told by Steve Lankton. I knew the story was about someone whose name began with an M and I couldn't remember it, and I could never find the exact source because I had heard it on tape. Julie was the one who told me its source. I told that story many, many times in therapy. It's an example of how you can use metaphor to bring up states which may need to be cleared for a client. The states it brings up for most people are sadness, grief, and other emotions that are involved in letting go and moving on with one's life. I used it quite a bit with clients before I ever introduced it into a training context.

The "Say Good-bye" metaphor is also an example of how to install strategies at the unconscious level. There was the "three-pile" strategy as well as saying "Good-bye." The three pile loop was nested inside "going inside the attic," to support on-going unconscious processing and conscious amnesia. All this is anchored within the phrase "**Say Good-bye.**" To handle the ecology of the effects which can come up with this metaphor, I followed it up with the third metaphor.

The third metaphor concerning the ritual burning of trees is a less effective metaphor but follows the same theme. It offers the opportunity for the listener to run the strategy of finding what is "unhealthy" and then decide how much they want to generalize the change so that it is ecological. It also provides the image of burning and transformation, and leads them to focus on what they want in the future. This metaphor was also set up to reframe loss or death and see it within a bigger picture. (Maybe you are thinking, "Yeah, isn't that obvious—I already knew that." If you are thinking something like that, then you have just experienced why it's generally not a good idea to explain metaphors!) This metaphor is anchored with the repetitive phrase to communicate: **Nothing really dies—it's just transformed; the change is natural,** which becomes the anchor for the entire piece.

Working with metaphor is truly a creative, collaborative process which will keep your therapy with your clients and, yes, yourself, fresh and evolving. As an intervention, it supports the process Bateson called "learning to learn,"[17] which is the development of adaptive action, or what some people call recursion. It's the idea of teaching the hungry person how to fish instead of just giving them the fish. Metaphor allows the client to structure and process information via comparison in terms of sameness and difference. This is a basic <u>meta</u>program. By the way, we're not just talking psychology here. According to Bateson,[18] this type of process is found throughout biology and is the basis of evolution. That's why he said, **"It becomes evident that metaphor is not just pretty poetry . . . it is in fact the logic upon which the biological world had been built . . . and the organizing glue of the world of mental process."**[19] In fact, the fundamental matrix of the human brain is metaphoric,[20] so why not use it? . . . And you thought we were just telling stories. Those old-time storytellers had it right. They really knew what was a <u>meta</u> for!

Chapter 10

Metaphorical Intervention: Is It Real Or Just A . . . ?

Editor's Notes: In this chapter, the trainers allude to the reason why Erickson was so effective in therapy, even though some people thought he was only "talking story." He would carry on a "normal" conversation and establish anchors for each of the resourceful states during the casual conversation. He would then fixate the client's attention in some way and briefly discuss the problem as he fired off the anchors while they were in trance. He was both subtle and brilliant.

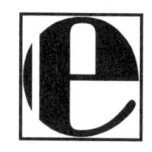

At this point in the training (the fourth day), the seminar participants are in rather profoundly altered states. Trance has become second nature as has communicating with their unconscious minds. Many of them report that this seminar brought things together for them and answered questions they had about hypnosis while increasing their confidence level. One of the "meta" outcomes of the training was to remove some of the mystique from hypnosis so the participants would feel ease and comfort in their work with clients. The Hypnotic Dream Induction further installed the processes learned earlier in the chapter and served as a vehicle to transfer the transformation that had occurred into their future. Note the effect of closing the loops from previous sections.

Question to the reader: What effect will having read this book have on your life?

In this section, we're going to integrate all of the preceding information which *you've been learning*. First, we're going to cover the Metaphorical Intervention, which we believe is one of the basic ways in which Erickson worked during the latter part of his career. This is a structure which we modeled from some of his published transcripts and tapes[1,2,3] and to our knowledge, it's not a pattern which is taught <u>explicitly</u> in NLP or Ericksonian Hypnosis. It is possible, however, to recognize it as something which many effective communicators do unconsciously when presenting information. Later in this section, we'll also outline our version of the Hypnotic Dream Intervention which has been used by many hypnotherapists (Ericksonian and Traditionalists alike).[4,5,6] We have used this intervention frequently with a great deal of success. We wanted to include it because most people agree that dreams are real while you're dreaming them and become metaphorical when you wake up . . . or is it the other way around? . . . . . . Either way, it's a lot like life!

The Metaphorical Intervention

1. Elicit client's present state and outcome.

2. Determine which resources/automatic processes would move the client from the present state to the outcome.

3. Tell the metaphors.

4. Anchor each metaphor auditorily.

5. Repeat Steps 3 and 4 until you have activated resources and notice indications of trance.

6. Do a formal, or more obvious, trance induction and fire the anchors for the metaphors.

7. Do the Posthypnotic Suggestion Protocol (from Chapter Eight).

As mentioned earlier, this interview is really an integration of the entire training. First, you'll get a general statement of your client's problem and outcome. You can casually ask about any hobbies and interests they have. Their areas of interest will give you ideas about which metaphors to use as resources. Once you elicit the problem, you can also ask yourself: "What resources or automatic processes would resolve this issue? What abilities are inherent in the problem that can be translated into hypnotic processes?" (Notice we're not doing a formal trance induction right now, which is different from the other formats we covered earlier.)

Next, begin the metaphors. You want to use these to illustrate points which are germane to moving the client from the present state to the outcome state. You can make a general statement about the point or ask a rhetorical question and then illustrate it with a metaphor. (Note: An example of this occurred earlier when we explained how metaphors work. We said that virtually anything can be an effective metaphor to the extent that a context is created wherein the client finds meaning in what is offered. We asked, "Why do metaphors work and exactly how do they work?" Then we told the story about the client with the Kleenex. We made a few general statements, asked a rhetorical question to set the context, and then told the story.)

While you're telling the metaphors, you're pacing the client and gradually modeling the physiology of trance. You don't need to mention "conscious" or "unconscious" explicitly to induce trance, as you did in Conscious-Unconscious Dissociation. You're just telling a story which evokes examples of automatic processing or naturally occurring hypnotic phenomena. It's that simple.

At the appropriate point in each story, i.e., the punch line or the statement of the theme, auditorily anchor each story with a word or a phrase and with a set of voice analogs (voice tone, tempo, timbre, locus, pitch, volume, etc.). Continue telling metaphors and anchoring them while building the necessary resources. The goal is to "light up" the neural networks so everything is in place, even if all the resources aren't needed. When an artist decides to paint a picture, she has her whole pallet of colors available to her. She may only use a few of them, but the others are there in case they're needed. Creativity and calibration are the keys.

At this point, it's time to formally induce trance. Notice that we're calling this the formal trance induction. More accurately, we're just being more obvious about inducing trance. Begin by recapping the reason for the therapy and also reviewing the problem and outcome, while further dissociating their conscious and unconscious functioning. After the client is in a sufficient trance, use anchors from the earlier metaphors. Then finish the trance with the posthypnotic suggestion protocol from Chapter Eight.

Group Demonstration

(Note: The numbers indicated throughout the demo refer to the steps outlined in the Metaphorical Intervention on page 184.)

1. So all of you want to be exquisite Ericksonian hypnotherapists, do you not? (Audience answers "yes.") Very good. And when you leave here you want to utilize these skills so that you, too, can produce elegant change, right? (Audience

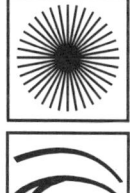

answers "yes.") Very good. And your internal representation about doing this well is a strong one with a compelling, positive kinesthetic, is it not? (Audience answers "yes.") Excellent.

1. And while you're very congruent about this now, there may be times in the future, albeit few and far between, when you might not be completely sure of your abilities, skills, etc. Since you are advanced in your understanding of hypnosis, there's no reason for us to remind you that when you're not sure of yourself it probably has something to do with an overactive conscious mind. In which case when you do remember this, you'll laugh to yourself and go immediately into trance. Trance is a wonderful way to experience life and sometimes we experience life more clearly when we observe the lives of others...

3. There was once a woman, whom I did not know personally, who went to a meet with a rishi master... Do you all know what a rishi is? A rishi is a seer, one who can see the Truth in all. This woman, who had travelled a long distance, went to the rishi master and told him of her purpose. "Sir, I have pursued many directions in my life. I have studied a number of disciplines and I have come to an important decision. I now know that what I want most of all is to learn to draw a perfect circle. I understand that you are a learned man and that you know and understand many things. I have heard that you know how to draw perfect circles and I wondered if you would draw one for me?"

The rishi master silently studied the woman before responding. She was not unlike the others who had preceded her with the same type of question, and she seemed quite sincere in this pursuit. In his humble manner he answered, "I would be honored." He went to a special glass case and removed an exquisite, black calligraphy pen and proceeded to draw a perfect circle. She was struck by the simple beauty of what he had produced and remarked, "That is a perfect circle. I don't think that I can do that. Will you teach me how to do that?" He responded to her request with a question: "How long have you been drawing your circles?" She said, "Four months, I've been practicing circles."

He then asked her to draw a circle. Making a deliberate effort to get it just right, she drew her circle. And her circle looked a lot like these ordinary circles; it wasn't really perfect. He said, "Ah, for months you've been drawing these circles and you're not quite sure you can draw a perfect circle. How long do you think it took me to draw a perfect circle?" "I'm not sure." "Forty years. Forty years to draw a perfect circle and you in four months have drawn a very, very good circle, but you're not yet __sure it's good enough__ ..... So, madam, if I am to make this trip worthwhile for you, I must say that if you keep chasing perfection, you'll be living your life in circles .... rather than __being sure__ .... of what you have drawn ... __in life__." The room became silent and all that reverberated within it was the twinkle in his eyes.

3. At the same time, down by the pier there was a particular boat about ten

to fifteen feet from the edge of the pier. It was loaded with many passengers. A young man, seeing the boat, checked his watch and thought, "Oh no, I'm not going to make it!" So he started running toward it at a very brisk pace. He wanted to catch the boat so he could make it on board. He ran the whole way over to the edge of the pier and finally he was close enough to the boat and he jumped right into it, landing inside the main cabin. He had made it. He sat down, and breathing heavily from all the effort, he took a very deep breath and finally relaxed.

(To audience) You know what it's like when your conscious mind thinks you're not going to make it, and then when you do there's that overwhelming sense of relief and you just relax? . . . As he's beginning to relax he hears a faint voice that becomes louder coming from inside the cabin . . . . ."That's right, just *relax* . . . . it's never too late . . . ." As the boatmaster emerges from the cabin and continues, "So you might as well *relax now* since you worked so hard to get on board. We were just coming in to dock. If you would have *relaxed and waited* a little longer, we would have picked you up!"

3. I actually went to my first hypnosis seminar when I was twenty-four years old, and it's the first time in my life where I remember having a spontaneous visual image. I saw a very vivid picture in my mind's eye and I was aware I was seeing it. (To audience) I don't know if that ever happened to you? Do you remember the first time you knew you were seeing pictures inside your head? At that time of my life, I was in one of those career "indecision" periods. I was having a "midlife crisis" early at age twenty-four!

I couldn't decide if I should go to law school, stay in family therapy, or do something else entirely different. So I used this as an issue in one of our exercises. I thought to myself, "*Hey, it's not going to get much safer than this, so if the opportunity's here, you might as well take it.*" I presented my dilemma of indecision to my unconscious mind and I didn't have a clue about what to expect. Almost immediately I received a response. (To audience) It's like you're in total indecision and you don't realize when you're unconscious . . . is in deciding what you really want . . . . in a moment's notice, you're in decision and through it before you know it.

"It's a picture," I realized. I saw a picture of the most vivid candy store I could ever imagine. (To audience) Do you remember penny candy stores? Maybe from when you were a kid or your parents were kids? The whole store glistened and every piece of penny candy glistened with a golden hue. Everything looked so pure and so clean. When I saw that, I heard inside my head, "Whatever you do . . . . . whatever you do . . . **it'll be okay**. Whatever you want . . . you can have . . . it'll be okay. **Whatever you do, it really will be okay**." Wow! That picture changed the course of my life because it really was **okay**.

3. I don't think there were any mangos in the candy store . . . (To audi-

ence) . . . by the way have you ever eaten a mango? If you haven't, then you may have heard of them. A mango is a sweet tropical fruit, about the size of a large avocado, with the consistency of a peach but with a flavor of its own. Very unique. One day a young man came home from his work and, upon walking into his courtyard, he found his uncle laboring in the hot sun. He approached his uncle and asked him what he was doing. "Well, I'm planting these seedlings." "What type of seedlings are they, uncle?" "Mangos, my son." "And how many are you planting?" "Ten in all."

"But uncle, do we have enough room in this small courtyard for ten mango trees?" "Yes, my son, I will see to it that they all fit." "Well, surely they will bear lots of fruit." "Thank you for your kind thoughts . . . I too hope they bear much fruit." "Uncle," the nephew asked patiently, "how long does it take for a mango tree to bear fruit?" "Twelve years, my son." "And how old are you now?" "I am ninety." "Uncle, I don't understand, why would you go to all the work of planting these mango trees now, if there's a chance you won't be here when they bear fruit?"

"Well, my young nephew, most likely you will be right and I will be in God's hands by the time they mature . . . but you see, all of my life I have eaten from mango trees which others have planted. Those trees will take twelve years until they mature. The comfort that I have is that other people will then be able to eat from the mango trees which I have planted. I'm not doing this for me, I'm *doing it for the others* so they can enjoy the fruits as I have for all my years. *I take comfort . . . . in knowing . . . . I'm doing it for others.*"[7]

6. So while your conscious mind is considering whatever it is . . . particularly since this is a training in trance . . . . . . Your unconscious mind has been very actively integrating both verbal and nonverbal information to support . . . you're learning hear what's next . . . . unless the conscious mind says "Never mind . . . . ." and you don't consciously because your unconscious will do it's part . . . while you go deeply into trance . . . and the best trances are those which you allow your unconscious to create without knowing it's happening.

6. Now, most of you are already intimately familiar with what it's like for you to be in a trance. How <u>do</u> you know when you're in trance? As you're positioned in the way you are, doing what you're doing at this moment . . . How would you know if **you're in a trance**? Does your breathing slow down the deeper you go into trance? Do your eyes want to blink a few more times before they gently rest . . . closed? And for some of you will it be the right hand, or the one that's left over there, that will easily, but unconsciously, lift to signal how comfortably you go into trance. And for others of you never mind that suggestion and just go deeper into trance as you experience those sensations inside . . . .

6. Thinking back to earlier . . . and I'm not sure now, when or really even if it will occur, but there may be a day after you leave here . . . . because this training in trance is drawing to a close, maybe tomorrow, the day after that, or maybe even several days later, you'll be working with someone, perhaps a client, and you won't even be thinking about perfect circles but you may stop and question yourself, "Am I _sure_ I did that ***well enough***?" "Did I do that technique, or that metaphor or that session well enough to help that person?" "Did I do it the way I should have or the way Erickson would have?"

6. And I don't know about you, it's taken me a number of years to get to this point and I'm still working on it . . . . because there may be the times when your conscious mind rushes to conclusions about how well you do things . . . even at the risk of going overboard in your efforts and not trusting . . . . the funniest thing is you'll only be tempted to do that until you realize just how much better it feels to ***relax and wait until it's really time*** . . . to be ***sure it's good enough*** . . . . and knowing that ***you relax more fully now***. It's really just a matter of timing. Because, however you do it, the choice really is yours. No one can make those decisions for you and, besides, any way you do it, it's ***going to be okay***. All the choices you could possibly make are okay choices. You know why? Because when you make choices for yourself with the full intention of sharing the fruits with others, you'll be okay. By the way, your work will always have a positive impact if you ***take comfort*** . . . in knowing . . . . ***you're doing it for others***. Keep that in mind whenever you work with someone.

7. You've all had the opportunity to spend this time in the training . . . in trance and as your conscious and unconscious minds know trance is a wonderful way to experience life. Did you ever wonder what it would be like if all of life was just a trance?

7. Because consciously you probably weren't thinking about a time in the future when you might feel like you're running in circles and when you're not ***sure*** that ***everything you're doing is good enough***, and your conscious mind might jump to conclusions until you remember how ***easy it is to relax and wait***. It's all a matter of timing. ***Everything will be okay as long as you do it for others. You can take comfort in that.*** And then you will certainly be an exquisite Ericksonian Hypnotherapist!

7. See, the great thing is you're not taking notes right now, and you probably remember from your school days how easy it is to forget what you haven't written down. Forgetting easily works with grocery lists, particularly if the list is only in your head. Once when John forgot something at the store and asked if he should go back, I said, "It's okay, you can forget it; we have all we need."

7. Because the next time you do go into a trance, you can enjoy it for what it is . . . a naturally occurring state . . . your state . . . the inner state running

through your United States . . . and that will allow you to go even deeper the next time . . . by the way, did you know that smiling to yourself will deepen a trance?

7. Now I wonder exactly how much your conscious and unconscious minds appreciate their level of cooperation with one another? It is fun to be in the flow of life and have things go your way every once in a while . . . and certainly you know who you have to thank for that . . . do you not? That's right, your conscious and you're unconscious, and you are . . . . so you may want to recognize them in some way that lets them know just how much you appreciate their increased cooperation with one another, so that they only surprise and delight you more in the future memories to come.

I like mangos, don't you? Meredith, you haven't had one? I hope someday you get to enjoy one: they're delicious!

Analysis of The Metaphor Intervention

As you're continuing to reorient and integrate all you're learning at the unconscious level, let's take this opportunity for some conscious analysis. We'll go through each of the major steps of the intervention. First, we should say that there are some things on which we won't comment, particularly the hypnotic languaging and the more artistic parts of the work. We'll limit our analysis to the "bare bones" of the steps pertinent to the intervention.

• *General statement of present state and outcome*

Because we did this with you, we used the general outcomes you had for coming to this training: to become exquisite Ericksonian hypnotherapists who are able to utilize these skills to produce elegant change. At the onset of the intervention, tag questions were used to create a "yes" set, to make sure the internal representation was strong and compelling.

• *Determine the resources/automatic processes that would move toward the outcome*

The questions to ask to get this information are very similar to those in the reframing section (when you were setting a particular theme). If you're dealing with a "problem," then you want to consider what positive abilities are inherent in the problem which would also be common to achieving the outcome. This will give you information about which "automatic processes" you want to activate and redirect. Examining the outcome or the client's stated purpose for the therapy will give you some obvious clues about which resources need to be mobilized. Finally, if you found out about hobbies and interests, these too could be revivified in the next phase.

The metaphors you just experienced were geared toward attributes, states, strategies, beliefs, and values which would tend to support your learning and development as a hypnotherapist.

• *Tell the metaphors and anchor them auditorily*

In this section, there were four metaphors which I used to communicate and anchor the resources. The rishi metaphor begins as a pacing metaphor. It paces the student-teacher relationship and the need for instant perfection which many folks may have. As the story continues, more hypnotic language is used. There's an interesting juxtaposition of the concepts of perfection and running in circles. Anchored to this is the reassurance "It's good *enough*" and "**Be sure in life.**"

The second metaphor (about the person running to catch the boat) paces what happens when we want too much too quickly, particularly if our conscious mind thinks we're not doing something well enough. Pressure from our conscious mind can distort our perception to the point that we don't know whether we're coming or going. The attitude suggested is, "You're going to make it one way or another; it's just a matter of time so '**Relax.**'" "Relax" is the primary anchor.

The "mid"-life crisis metaphor had a number of features in it. It dealt with indecision within an ongoing process and its resolution. It gave the unconscious mind a specific strategy for assisting the conscious mind as well as communicating, "*Whatever you do, it really will be okay*," which was the anchor.

The final story was the story about the old man and the mango tree. It was the most effective of the sequence. It couples the feelings you develop toward the old man with comfort and with doing things for other people. It's a metaphor designed to communicate values and a more spiritual message. The anchors are, "*Take comfort . . .* **in knowing . . . in doing it for others.**"

• *Induce a formal trance and fire anchors*

Next, I began the "formal induction" which, at this point in this training, uses very brief references to trance since you're all great hypnotic subjects. Then it was just a matter of firing off the anchors sequentially in relation to future performance: "Because consciously you probably weren't thinking about a time in the future when you might feel like you're running in circles and

192 TRAINING TRANCES

when you're not _sure_ that _everything you're doing is good enough_, and your conscious mind might even think of rushing ahead until you remember how easy it is _relax and wait_. It's all a matter of timing. _Everything will be okay as long as you do it for others. You can take comfort in that_. And then you will certainly be an exquisite Ericksonian Hypnotherapist!" This then becomes quite powerful because revivifying the metaphors in another trance amplifies the learnings.

- ## *Posthypnotic suggestion protocol*

After everything else you experienced, this is the icing on the cake. It seals off everything and at the same time gives you another opportunity to reinforce the learnings. It's a great way to end.

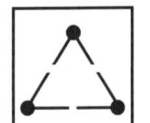

Metaphorical Intervention

1. General statement of client's problem and outcome.

2. Determine what resources/automatic processes would move the client from the present state to the outcome.
Use the same thought process for setting the theme of the therapy.

3. Metaphors:
   a. general statement of point. (Optional—We noted that Erickson often did this, but many time it's more effective to go to b.)
   b. metaphor or analogy:
      (1) nonverbal pace and lead (modeling trance).
      (2) evoke examples of automatic processing.
      (3) no mention of conscious-unconscious explicitly.

4. Anchor each story auditorily with a phrase or word and a specific set of auditory analogs.

5. Repeat Steps 3 and 4 until you have activated resources and notice indications of trance.

6. Formal, or just more obvious, trance induction:
   a. Conscious-Unconscious Dissociation.
   b. induce catalepsy (for later use, if you like).
   c. fire auditory anchors in relation to the present state.

> *Continued ...*
>
> 7. Posthypnotic suggestion protocol (from Chapter Eight):
>   a. trance
>   b. new behaviors
>   c. amnesia
>   d. trance
>   e. self-appreciation

This is a neat intervention. This is where we've been headed the whole time. So find a willing listener and .... go for it!

Do the exercise

How many of you noticed it was surprisingly easier than you thought it would be, even though there might have been some moments when you thought, "What am I going to say?" (A number of people raise their hands.)

When we went around to the groups, some said that after they elicited the problem and the outcome, they realized that the metaphors which they had prepared (about learning) didn't seem to be appropriate to the context. So they "had" to *trust* their *unconscious mind* and flow with whatever metaphors they developed on the spot.

This is one of the ways in which metaphors are created. Many times, we've had the experience of working with a particular client and saying something "off the cuff" which was very effective. We'll make a note of it and consider all the other situations in which the story would be useful. Then we'll begin to *develop it*. This is an easy way to build a repertoire of metaphors for use in a variety of situations. Case studies also work well for this purpose. In our research of Erickson's work, it becomes apparent that he had twenty or thirty metaphors which he used in different settings, modifying them based on the context and his observation of the listener(s).

The "garage" metaphor which we used to open the training began as a side comment a number of years ago. All I wanted to do was set an anchor for the word "inside." I recalled Erickson's guest house also being referred to as a reconverted garage.[8] I mentioned that Dr. Erickson would do all of his teaching "inside the garage." I liked the idea of a garage better than a guest house, because of the obvious associations: a place to do work, to repair or fix things, and where things are often stored. Most people have their own memories of playing or working in a garage which makes it a fairly universal metaphor. After awhile, my unconscious mind began coming up with other ideas and the metaphor evolved into one of activating archetypes of the unconscious mind. It continued to evolve from training to training through the reactions of students and our response to them. Eventually it took on a life of its own. Each time we do a metaphor, we make new connections as new things come out of our mouths—it becomes an active, creative process between the speaker and the listener.

The Hypnotic Dream Induction

We are going to close this training in trance with our version of the Hypnotic Dream Induction. This version is an amalgam of several versions which we've read and enjoyed.[9,10] For the most part, we attribute this particular induction to Erickson's work with a sprinkling of ideas from Stephen Gilligan.

In my first career I did regular therapy, and in my second one I did Hypnosis and NLP. Very early on in my second career, I was working with this woman who wanted to quit smoking, but she had "some other things" she needed to "straighten out."

She had been in a number of abusive relationships. At that time, she was in a relationship with a man who was emotionally abusive and she admitted she was addicted to the relationship. While they didn't live together, she still could not find an easy way to end the relationship. She insisted that he was not threatening to harm her and wouldn't if she decided to end the relationship.

When closing the first couple of sessions with her, I made generative suggestions that her unconscious could complete the work in her dreams and/or keep things on hold so she could give them her complete attention in therapy. This would assist her in functioning well throughout the day. After these initial sessions, she began making changes.

As the sessions progressed, it sometimes seemed like we wouldn't get very far in the appointments themselves. With a few minutes left in each session, I suggested that, before going to sleep each night, she repeat the following suggestion, "Ask your unconscious mind while you sleep soundly and dream tonight to go ahead and do X,Y, and Z to the extent that it is comfortable for you." She'd come in the following week, and of course we wouldn't get very far in the session, so I would be left with giving her the same suggestion again. I soon realized that this was the therapy. She was making all of her changes in her dreams.

On several occasions, she said she awakened with strong positive feelings like security, love, and confidence (very uncharacteristic for her) with no understanding of why they were there or to what they were connected. These feelings often stayed with her throughout the day and would be renewed each night. She had one or two "bad days" over the course of a week, just enough to keep her engaged in therapy so she would "get to the bottom of things."

The other thing which usually happened closer to the next therapy session was that she would awaken with a thought or a picture, often abstract but very vivid and persistent. This was slightly unsettling to her, as she was not prone to a lot of analysis. She usually said something like "John, I woke up and had this thought. I don't know what this means, but I thought I better tell you about it." These things usually turned out to be very relevant to her therapy.

Although it took me awhile, I eventually realized what her unconscious mind was up to! She'd come in and we'd induce trance. While she was in trance, we talked about what she was going to do in her dream that night and that would be the session. So I didn't even bother doing "regular" therapy or "NLP" therapy with her, because she wasn't doing the changework during the sessions anyway.

The outcome of her dreamwork was quite positive. She ended the relationship, lost weight, and quit smoking. I learned a lot from her therapy and began using dreams as a resource for trancework and vice versa. It's easy because the dream state and the trance state are virtually the same; what is done in one state will often quite nicely continue into the other state, particularly if it's suggested. It all becomes the client's therapy, injected with the meaning from their dreams. For the most part, it keeps the therapist out of the interpretation game and puts them into the <u>integration frame</u>. The outline on the next page provides the flexibility of doing "dreamwork" in the session, as well as setting up night dreams.

Hypnotic Dream Induction

1. Elicit present state and outcome state.
   • establish a "yes set."

2. Dissociate: Problem <————————> Solution
   Conscious <————————> Unconscious

   • use auditory anchors, words, and your physiology to create dissociation.

3. Unconscious mind ————————>Middle of (K)Nowhere

4. Sleep ————> Dreaming ————> Thought

5. Hypnotic dream with catalepsy (repeat as often as necessary).

6. Thought ————> Dreaming ————> Sleep

7. Middle of (K)Nowhere ————> Unconscious mind

Instructions Leading Into A Demonstration

It might be fun to do this one totally content-free. The therapist doesn't need to know what the specific issue is, although the client does. As the therapist, all you have to do is look at the client and say, "You have this thing you would like to improve or change, do you not?" They nod "yes." You say, "Great, that's excellent . . . and there's probably something which you want to be doing differently . . . . . or to improve . . . . . and you do, don't you?" "Yesssss."

Conscious-Unconscious Dissociation

The next step is the same approach we utilized in the Hypnotic Interview and in the Metaphorical Intervention. Use auditory anchors so you have your conscious mind voice and you have your unconscious mind voice. Begin the Conscious-Unconscious Dissociation relative to the problem and the solution. (You may want to refer to Chapter Four.) Gradually begin spending less time talking to the conscious mind and more time talking to the unconscious mind.

Group Demonstration

You can probably imagine, consciously, how that will go . . . *while your unconscious mind is doing something else that prepares you to do this . . . . Now,* you may feel a little anxious or un . . . **sure of yourself.** How can you expect that you'll be completely comfortable the first time you do this? But *your unconscious mind knows about all the other "first" times when you did far better than you expected. It knew what to do then and it* **knows what to do now,** *even though you don't think you do. It has stored all of your memories and knows how to do things automatically,* so consciously you can focus on whatever you deem important or even better, what will **make this an enjoyable experience** for you . . . . without the slightest awareness that *your unconscious can work independently, on its own . . . . . . and what will be the most effective means to prepare you to use this information and make whatever changes you want to make? I don't know and why should I? . . . . . when your unconscious can do it so much more quickly and in a way that best suits your total personality.*

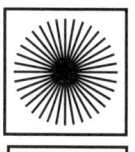

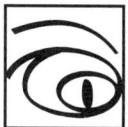

Middle of (k)nowhere

. . . . . *And it's this spirit of cooperation that can free up your conscious mind to wa(o)nder . . . . wherever it wants,*
nowhere in particular . . . .
(k)nowhere you've been,
(k)nowhere you are,
(k)nowhere you're going . . . . . .

Whereas your unconscious mind can float . . . . as mind and not as a body and get to the heart of the matter . . . the center of it all . . . .

The middle of (k)nowhere . . . and you do (k)nowhere . . . just floating . . .
(k)nowhere you've been,
(k)nowhere you are,
(k)nowhere you're going,
in the middle of (k)nowhere . . . . It's a lot like sleeping . . . .

Sleep

. . . . . *And when you're asleep, you're asleep. Nowhere in particular.* **Just sleep.** *And the wonderful thing about sleep is that, as you're sleeping, your body rests . . . . . . it can* **heal** *. . . . . . because it knows how to heal naturally while you sleep so as to allow your body to regenerate and rejuvenate . . . . .*

Dreams
..... And while you're sleeping **you can dream** ..... *You dream, I dream, everybody dreams. And in a dream you don't have to know **you're in a dream** when you are. Nowhere in particular in a dream is the best place to be in a dream* ... *And the wonderful thing about dreams is that they can* **have lasting, profound, and beneficial effects which can stay with you for the rest of your life** .... *and sometimes you don't even know that you're dreaming when you are dreaming. Because while you're dreaming you can easily translate any external sounds or stimuli into your dream world. Any sound, any touch is easily trans-lated into your dream* ...... *Now, we don't know what kinds of dreams you'll have* .....

Thought
.... *But the one thing that is really fantastic about dreaming* .... *is that all that happens while* **you're dreaming** ... *is thought. You're your thought and everything and everyone is your thought* .... *and you know how natural thought is* ...... *It's so easy to think* .... *without even thinking about it* . .... *no matter* .... **It's so easy to think** ...... *about* **whatever you want.** *They're just thoughts* ...... *your thoughts* ...... *You can make thoughts of whatever you want. At the level of thought there is no time, no place, but now. You are free to do whatever you can think that supports your well-being and those around you* .....

Hypnotic dream and catalepsy
(Provide a suggestion that you will reach over and pick up their arm. Pick up their arm and establish catalepsy. Suggest that the arm can go down as quickly as it takes for a dream to begin and have it end with the hand touching the leg. Repeat this to chunk the work or to facilitate different perspectives or different dreams.)

.... *So I don't know just how you'd like to use this dream, (reach over and lift their arm which is now cataleptic) but I do know* **you can have a dream only as quickly as that arm goes back down to your lap** ..... **a full, complete dream that will satisfy your outcome** *in a way you would have never dreamed of before. That's right, allow that arm to come down* .....

(If you want, once their arm reaches their lap, you know what you do, don't you? You pick it back up again.)

..... *I'd like you to have the same dream but with different characters this time so* **you can experience things from a different point of view** *from having different characters so that you solidify that outcome to an even greater ex-*

tent. And as the arm goes down and touches the leg, and the dream has ended . . .

(If you want, pick up their arm again.)

. . . Have a dream again, but this time with a different plot, so you can appreciate how well you can adapt to unexpected and different things that can happen in different ways and enjoy changing with life . . . . .

Thought
. . . . . Since everything is a thought, it's easy to think you can have more dreams than what you've just dreamed now . . . . later on while you sleep . . . . . Anything is possible at the level of thought . . . It's easy to think . . . . . and everything that has ever been created in your world began with a thought . . .

Dream
*. . . . . And all of this can happen inside of a dream . . . . **You'll have several dreams each night** . . . . . Whether you know it or not . . . . . dreams can have lasting, profound beneficial effects that can stay with you for the rest of your life . . . . . You can dream each night to consolidate your learnings and to creatively find solutions . . . . . . You can generate and practice new ways of thinking, ways of being the person you have dreamed you want to be and become it. Because just as . . . while you're dreaming **your dream will become a trance-lator** for any external sounds or stimuli which are incorporated into your dream world. You can when you awaken and translate what has occurred in your dream world to your external world in ways which support you and others.*

Sleep
. . . . . While you're dreaming, your unconscious mind continues to make all those chemical changes you need to make so you feel refreshed and alert . . . . because that's really what sleeping is for, to allow your body to relax . . . to experience deep rest . . . (k)nowhere in particular . . . . . naturally . . . . .

Middle of (k)nowhere
. . . . . And I don't know how soon you'll begin to wander once again in the middle of you (k)nowhere . . . . that's right
(k)nowhere in particular,
(k)now where you've been,
*until **you are ready** . . . . .*
(k)nowhere you are,
***(k)nowwhere you're going,** that's really all that matters.*

Unconscious-conscious reintegration
..... *So as your unconscious mind begins to* **solidify and crystalize those changes** *that it's made, your conscious mind might actually begin to enjoy clearly listening in a way it hadn't before. And I don't know how much thought you've given to future times, future changes that will be a direct result of what it is that you've just done. That may well be a matter for your unconscious mind to know and for you to find out! Because what is most important is your own appreciation for how well your* **unconscious and conscious mind cooperate and can work together in ways which make you one-of-a-kind person** *... who is increasingly more conscious of yourself and those around you.*

Do the exercise

Discussion

Do you have any questions about how the hypnotic dream induction works? Incidentally, the catalepsy is totally optional. You can just ask them to begin a dream and signal when it's done, without using catalepsy.

CHRIS: My partner seemed to come out of trance immediately after the first dream when his hand touched his leg. All I did was just lift the arm again, and as soon as I let go of it, it was cataleptic.

It's okay if he comes back out because then you're fractionating the trance. It's fine if the client comes back outside; just assist them in going back into trance again. You can also point out that people often wake up between dreams.

AUDIENCE: I couldn't seem to elicit catalepsy from my partner. The arm was a dead weight.

It is possible at times for a person to go so deeply into trance that they whistle right past catalepsy. You may lift their arm and it's very heavy. You'll want to utilize whatever the person does and just weave it right into what you're doing. You could suggest that in a moment, the dream can begin when they feel that hand hit their leg. It will be like how your body jerks just before you fall in a deep sleep ...... now. You act like it's what you expected and you always expect the unexpected. Like Erickson said, "You can pretend anything and master it."[11] Observe your person, watch everything they do and incorporate it into what you're doing with them.

AUDIENCE: When would it be useful to do the hypnotic dream induction?

We've used variations of this extensively in therapy. We use dreams a lot whenever time is running out at the end of a session. We would even do a dream induction like we just did, and within the "dream" phase of the induction, we provide a suggestion about having a dream later that night.

One of the wonderful things about doing dreamwork is that the person's conscious mind has every right to go ahead and deny the existence of a dream. It's perfect. With many people, as soon as you start to talk about dreams in any extensive way, you may not even have to suggest amnesia because of the current associations they have to their dreamlife. For example, if you have a person who doesn't believe that they dream, they can still have the dreams you've suggested and totally deny that they've ever had them.

If you have a person who remembers their dreams very well, they'll probably be able to tell you pieces of the dreams they had. When you suggest a dream, simply by saying the word "dream" you're going to fire off associations about a complex set of processes.[12] For some people, dreams mean doing things at night and never remembering them. Others place heavy, mystical significance on these nighttime activities.

We may also use it at the end of breakthrough sessions (a session around a specific life area which is approximately three hours on the first day and two or three hours on the following day). We write down all the major themes or learnings which the client experienced in the breakthrough session. Then we do a combination of this induction and the metaphorical induction and fire off all of the learnings inside of the dream induction. It's a nice finishing piece, particularly if someone has come from out of town to do therapy, because it creates momentum and generative possibilities for their return home.

This intervention is also useful with clients who naturally present their dreams as part of the therapy process. This is a great therapeutic induction to do with them because it makes use of an unconscious process (unless they are lucid dreamers) in which they're already interested. Just about anything done in trance can be done in dreams and vice versa.[13] If hypnogogic and hypnopompic states are included, then the client also has these powerfully creative and integrative states available. One would be hard pressed to make any substantial distinctions between hypnogogic/hypnopompic states and trance.[14] During these states, it's a great time to make self-suggestions. As far as we're concerned, the person's "dreamer" is their internal therapist. What's even better is that this therapist has evening hours! How many gifted therapists do you know who work the night shift every day of the week?

There are a couple of caveats when using dreams, or hypnogogic and hypnopompic states, in a deliberate way. If you're using the time just before you fall asleep to set up dreams, make sure you add something like, "<u>While I</u>

sleep soundly and dream . . . . . so I feel rested and refreshed when I awaken." Include this suggestion if you want to get a good night's sleep—otherwise your unconscious may help you to make whatever changes you've requested at the expense of a comfortable night's sleep. This suggestion gives the unconscious some guidelines in which to operate. Make your suggestion short and direct. Tell your unconscious mind what you would like it to do, but not specifically how you want it to do it. When you awaken, check in with the unconscious and notice if it is signaling you in any way. If it's not, let it go immediately and go about your day. Do expect that when you least expect it, something may come through.

A great thing is to put the hypnotic dream induction on tape and listen to it before you dream at night. At times, however, it's important to listen to the tape in the middle of the day and not before going to bed. I once made an extensive tape because I wanted to dream lucidly (where you wake up in the dream and know you're dreaming). I created these great inductions for myself, and the whole thing backfired. I listened to it four or five nights in a row, and it was the first time in my life that I didn't even remember any of my dreams. I realized that this was not working. As soon as I lightened up on myself, I started to remember my dreams again, and soon after that I began having lucid dreams.

So, this closes our section on the Hypnotic Dream Induction and the Metaphorical Intervention, and we're drawing near the close of this training in trance. There are a few loose ends . . . . .

Is this really a dream? Or is it just a . . . . . ?

Meanwhile, the student was waiting for the Master Woodcutter to tell him the second thing he needed to know to become a master. The time had come for the student's final task. He had really gotten to the point where the Master Woodcutter said, "**You are ready to be a master.**" He continued saying, "**To be a master you have to go out and apply what you've learned.**" The student thought deeply about what the master said. The Master Woodcutter then told him that tomorrow they would both get up with the sun, get their axes and head into the woods. Once in the woods they would identify what needed to be cut down and continue cutting until sunset. At sunset, they would see whose pile was the largest.

The student thought, "This is great!" He looked at the Master Woodcutter—who looked old, weathered, and thin now that he spent most of his time only telling stories—and felt a surge of adrenalin at the prospect of becoming a Master.

The next day came, and the Master Woodcutter walked out of his cabin with his axe. The student was waiting with his axe and together they walked out into the forest. They began chopping. They chopped and chopped and trees fell, splinters flew with the each crack of their axes. The piles grew. As the student strained to carry as much wood as he could to his pile, he looked over at the Master Woodcutter and saw the Master Woodcutter slowing down. In fact, he saw the Master Woodcutter stop and sit down, sort of slumped over. Totally inspired by this, the student thought to himself, "I'm young. I'm vital. I can do all this stuff. He's an old man, he can't keep up with me. He gave me all his knowledge, but it's my time now. I can do it. I know I can do it."

With this, the student kept chopping away at a feverish pace. Adrenalin. Motivation. Faster and faster. With each whack he made, his sweat flew through the air already filled with loud exhales and the cracking of splintering wood.

Hours passed, and he looked over and once again saw the Master Woodcutter stop, sit back down, and slump over with his back to the student. "I knew it was my time, I knew it was my time," the student thought and continued chopping away. Dusk approached, and with one last great burst of adrenalin, the student made his final charge for the finish. Sweat flying, hands blistering, forearms aching, he mustered every scrap of energy he had.

Again he noticed the Master Woodcutter sitting down just minutes before the student took down his last tree. The sun set behind the mountains, covering the woods with the night. All was quiet but for the breaking of twigs beneath the student's boots and the hoot of a distant owl. As he walked over to the Master Woodcutter, his heart still pumped wildly. His exhaustion gave way to relief and elation. He had given his all and with that thought, his eyes welled up. He wasn't quite sure why. All he knew was that he had cut more wood than he ever dreamed was possible. He knew he had done his very best.

"Now it's time to see," said the Master Woodcutter, arresting the student's reverie. The Master Woodcutter got out his big flashlight and shined the light over toward the student's pile. The student saw the huge pile of wood he had cut that day. He felt proud of what he had accomplished. Tangible results. He actually saw tangible results of what was done and what the training had produced.

The student stood and watched the beam of light move across the dark shadows of the trees in front of them, as the Master Woodcutter redirected the light to <u>his</u> pile . . . . . the Master Woodcutter was silent.

The student looked and couldn't believe his eyes. The Master Woodcutter's pile was even larger than his. He was awestruck in utter disbelief. The student looked at the Master Woodcutter and asked, "I don't get it. I just don't get it. How did you do it? I worked at a feverish pace for so long and you even had to stop. I don't get it. What were you doing?" The Master Woodcutter looked at him and answered, "I was sharpening my blade . . . . "

"And now you've learned the second thing that you need to know to be a Master Woodcutter:

There's always more to learn."

And what was the fourth key to doing Ericksonian work and being certifiable? As we said, there's always more to learn!

So as you go along your way, there will be many signs along the path of your progress. Remember to signal your intentions when you see the right signs. We certainly hope you enjoy many *driving trances* as you're moving toward all your destinations.

Driving trances are the most fun! They can **open your eyes** and make **you aware** of all the **new possibilities** along your way.

AND SO . . . . .

THIS IS THE END OF ONE DREAM THAT TWO PEOPLE LIVED . . .

ABOUT A TRAINING

. . . . . IN TRANCE . . . . .

. . . . . IN TRAINING . . . . .

NOW IT'S YOUR TURN . . . . .

End Notes

Chapter 1

1. George Miller, "The magical number seven, plus or minus two: some limits on our capacity for processing information," *Psychological Review* 63 (1956): 81-97.
2. Byron Lewis and R. Frank Pucelik, *Magic Demystified* (Portland, OR: Metamorphous Press, 1982), 7.
3. Wilder Penfield, *The Mystery of the Mind: A Critical Study of Consciousness and the Human Brain* (Princeton, NJ: Princeton University Press, 1975). This book summarizes Penfield's life's work in the area of memory. He reached these conclusions as early as the 1920s in his research on localization of memory and brain functioning.
4. Jeffrey Zeig, *A Teaching Seminar with Milton H. Erickson* (New York: Brunner/Mazel, 1980), 173.
5. Ibid.
6. Karl Pribram, *Languages of the Brain*, 5th Edition (Monterey, CA: Wadsworth Publishing, 1977). Also, Daniel Goleman, "Holographic Memory: Karl Pribram Interviewed by Daniel Goleman," Psychology Today 12, no. 9 (February 1979). It should be noted here that *we* are suggesting that memory is stored holographically throughout the *body*. We are basing this on later findings in neuropeptide research cited below in citation 7. Pribram confined his model to the *brain*. His earliest formulations of the holographic brain model were put forth in 1966.
7. Candace Pert, "The Chemical Communicators," in Bill Moyers, *Healing and the Mind* (New York: Doubleday, 1993), 178-181. Initial findings and later corroboration that neuropeptides are everywhere in the body occurred after Pribram's earlier work with the holographic model of the brain, when neuropeptides were thought to be located only in the brain. Therefore we're extending his holography model in light of the insight that neuropeptides are present throughout the body.
8. Benjamin Libet, "Unconscious cerebral initiative and the role of conscious will in voluntary action," *Behavioral and Brain Sciences* 8 (1985): 529-566.
9. B. J. Baars, *A Cognitive Theory of Consciousness* (Cambridge: Cambridge University Press, 1988).
10. Stephen and Carol Lankton, *The Answer Within: A Clinical Framework of Ericksonian Hypnotherapy* (New York: Brunner/Mazel, 1983), 6.
11. Benjamin Libet et al., "Subjective referral of the timing for a conscious sensory experience: A functional role for the somatosensory specific projection system in man," *Brain* 102, pt. 1 (March 1979): 193-224. For us,

this puts to rest any doubt about the importance of unconscious functioning in *everything* we do, even conscious processing. It also explains how and why we often attribute to our conscious mind much more than its fair share of functioning. If you want an extremely lucid account of this series of studies, read Fred Alan Wolf, *The Dreaming Universe* (New York: Simon & Schuster, 1994). He's using this research for slightly different purposes in his book, but he mentions the points we're making in this book.

12. Peter Brown, *The Hypnotic Brain* (New Haven, CT: Yale University Press, 1991), 135-136. Brown cites approximately ten different studies that he found to be "carefully designed," which had used "a variety of methodologies." From our review, this book is one of the more readable research-oriented books on hypnosis as a form of communication.

13. Stewart Hulse, James Deese, and Howard Egeth, *The Psychology of Learning*, 4th Edition (New York: McGraw-Hill, 1975), 330-331.

14. P. Lewicki, *Nonconscious Social Information Processing* (Orlando, FL: Academic Press, 1986), 220. This is nicely summarized in Brown, *The Hypnotic Brain*, 136.

15. Ibid.

16. Andre Weitzenhoffer, *The Practice of Hypnotism*, Vol. 2 (New York: John Wiley & Sons, 1989), 197. Both of these volumes are a must read for a number of reasons, most notably Weitzenhoffer's unique perspective. He is a scholar in the field of hypnosis and a contemporary of Erickson, capable of giving a balanced appraisal of the fact and the myth of Erickson and his work.

17. **Note:** There has been a lively debate in the field of hypnosis about whether hypnosis is a formal state or not. At this point, mainstream science recognizes three formal or "special" states: waking, sleeping, and dreaming. Our own experience and our review of recent literature leaves little doubt that hypnosis is, indeed, a state, although it may not be a "special state," as some have hypothesized. It is likely that as technology increases so will our ability to clarify this distinction. Incidentally, hypnosis suffers from the same plight as dreams. Some scientists argue that although we can measure rapid eye movement and other physiological parameters; and although subjects can report that they are dreaming, there is still no "scientific" evidence that dreaming exists. Imagine that!

18. J. Alan Hobson, *The Dreaming Brain: How the Brain Creates Both the Sense and the Nonsense of Dreams* (New York: Basic Books, 1988). The physiological mechanisms that Hobson and McCarley identify in their activation-synthesis hypothesis of dreaming may be quite similar to what happens in trance. There is increasing research into the biological and physiological actions associated with hypnosis. A literature review by Gabel ("The right hemisphere in imagery, hypnosis, rapid eye movement, sleep and dreaming: empirical studies and tentative conclusions," *Journal of Nervous and Mental Disease* 176, 323-331) indicates that, on the

whole, changes in lateralization of hemispheric activity occur in hypnosis and that these changes generally result in increased right hemispheric activity. According to Brown in *The Hypnotic Brain*, it might be more appropriate to say that there is inhibited left hemispheric EEG activity in hypnosis. Hypnosis is correlated with alpha and theta activity.

The limbic system seems to be active in the generation of any altered states. With a close connection between the cortex and the rest of the body the limbic system is in a pivotal position for integrating psychological and physiological functioning. Hypnosis is characterized by increased parasympathetic activity. Our anterior hypothalamus inhibits the reticular activating system and facilitates the release of cholinergic cells which slows our internal processes, making us less aware of our overall surroundings. According to DeBenedittis and Sironi, ("Arousal effects of electrical deep brain stimulation in hypnosis," *International Journal of Clinical and Experimental Hypnosis* 36, 96-106) during hypnosis there are two areas in the limbic system which appear to play important roles:

1. The hippocampus is largely responsible for the registration and retrieval of emotionally important memories, making sure they are available for comparison with the external world. The cells of the hippocampus are involved in chunking information that is being attended to in any given situation. It stimulates the processing of information and the comparison with existing knowledge. The overall neurological action of the hippocampus is inhibitory, and with hypnosis there is increased hippocampal activity.

2. The amygdala coordinates emotional states with the appropriate external objects. Its job is primarily excitatory, thereby stimulating externally oriented behavior. When you "wake up" and reorient from trance there is increased amygdal activity. (...And so it goes... This is just a piece of one layer of a multidimensional puzzle that may as likely be solved by a quantum physicist as a researcher in physiologically based sciences.)

19. D. Kripke and D. Sonnenschein, "A biologic rhythm in waking fantasy" in K. Pope and J. Singer, eds., *The Stream of Consciousness: Scientific Investigations into the Flow of Human Experience* (New York: Plenum Press, 1978), 321-332.
20. Ernest Rossi, *The Psychobiology of Mind-Body Healing* (New York: W.W. Norton, 1986). Also, see citation 21. This is where Rossi first published his hypothesis.
21. Ernest Rossi, "Hypnosis and ultradian cycles: A new state(s) theory of hypnosis?" *American Journal of Clinical Hypnosis* 25 (1982): 21-32.
22. Daniel Spiegel and Herbert Spiegel, "Hypnosis" in H. Kaplan and B. Sadock, eds., *Comprehensive Textbook of Psychiatry*, Vol. IV (Baltimore: Williams and Wilkins, 1985), 1389.
23. Jay Haley and Madeleine Richeport, *Milton H. Erickson, M.D.: Explorer in Hypnosis and Therapy* (videotape) (New York: Brunner/Mazel, 1993).

24. Richard Bandler, *Time for a Change* (Cupertino, CA: Meta Publications, 1993), 44. An earlier reference to this idea is in J. Grinder and R. Bandler, *TRANCE-formations* (Moab, UT: Real People Press), 13.
25. Milton Erickson, Ernest Rossi, and Sheila Rossi, *Hypnotic Realities* (New York: Irvington Publishers, 1976).
26. Ibid.
27. **Note:** Somnambulism is generally considered synonymous with deep trance, according to Crasilneck and Hall, *Clinical Hypnosis Principle and Applications*, 2nd Edition (Orlando: Grune & Stratton, 1985), 13. Signs of somnambulism include ability to open the eyes without affecting the trance, virtually complete amnesia, posthypnotic anesthesia and analgesia, age regression, posthypnotic positive and negative hallucination, and lip pallor. Our observation is that while in a somnambulistic trance, clients may have considerable difficulty speaking to the extent that they may actually have to lighten the trance a bit to talk. They are almost completely literal in their responses to suggestions and may often appear stuporous. We refer to somnambulists as those who will exhibit many of these signs with little or no training in hypnosis.
28. George Estabrooks, *Hypnotism* (New York: E.P. Dutton, 1943), 136. For a very complete collection and analysis of distribution studies done on hypnotic susceptibility using depth scales from 1930-1980, see: Andre Weitzenhoffer, *The Practice of Hypnotism*, Vol. 2 (New York: John Wiley & Sons, 1989), 168.
29. Andre Weitzenhoffer, *The Practice of Hypnotism*, Vol. 2 (New York: John Wiley & Sons, 1989), 186-187.

Chapter 2

1. Milton Erickson, *Healing in Hypnosis*, Ernest Rossi, Margaret Ryan and Florence Sharp, eds. (New York: Irvington Publishers, 1983), 20-21.
2. Ibid., 19-22.
3. George Estabrooks, *Hypnotism* (New York: E.P. Dutton, 1943), 136.
4. E. I. Banyai, I. Meszaros, and L. Csokay, "Interaction between hypnotist and subject: A social psychophysiological approach" (preliminary report) in *Modern Trends in Hypnosis*, D. Waxman, P. Mizra, M. Gibson, and M. Maker, eds. (New York: Plenum Press, 1985), 97-108.
5. Boris Sidis, *Psychology of Suggestion* (New York: Appleton & Co., 1898), 19-23. This book is not easy to get, but well worth the effort.
6. Milton Erickson, *Creative Choice in Hypnosis*, Ernest Rossi and Margaret Ryan, eds. (New York: Irvington Publishers, 1992), 152. Erickson's affinity toward indirection is peppered throughout many different papers, lectures, and books. This reference summarizes many of the others we've read: "In psychotherapy, it is always better to get things happening indirectly."

7. Peter Brown, *The Hypnotic Brain* (New Haven, CT: Yale University Press, 1991), 234.
8. Boris Sidis, *Psychology of Suggestion* (New York: Appleton & Co., 1898), 51-52.
9. Ibid.
10. Ibid., 23.
11. Peter Brown, *The Hypnotic Brain* (New Haven, CT: Yale University Press, 1991), 237.
12. L. J. Kirmayer, "Word magic and the rhetoric of common sense: Erickson's metaphors for mind," International *Journal of Clinical and Experimental Hypnosis* 36 (1988): 157-172.
13. E. I. Banyai, I. Meszaros, and L. Csokay, "Interaction between hypnotist and subject: A social psychophysiological approach" (preliminary report), in *Modern Trends in Hypnosis*, D. Waxman, P. Mizra, M. Gibson, and M. Maker, eds. (New York: Plenum Press, 1985), 97-108.
14. Milton Erickson, Ernest Rossi, and Sheila Rossi, *Hypnotic Realities* (New York: Irvington Publishers, 1976).
15. Milton Erickson, *Healing in Hypnosis*, Ernest Rossi, Margaret Ryan, and Florence Sharp, eds. (New York: Irvington Publishers, 1983), 27-28.
16. Ibid., 27, 42-43. A historical note to set the record straight. We took liberties in collapsing the time period from the time that the Ericksons arrived in Phoenix to the time they reached Hayward Avenue. It flows better with the themes of the metaphor. In 1948, Dr. and Mrs. Erickson moved to Arizona and lived on the grounds of Arizona State Hospital. About a year later, Erickson began his private practice in his home on Cypress Street. In 1970, they moved into the Hayward Avenue home with the guest house (the garage). The idea for the metaphor came after reading Jeffrey Zeig's book, *A Teaching Seminar with Milton H. Erickson*. We recall that the actual "garage" idea was developed after listening to Stephen Lankton, *Ericksonian Therapy*, wherein the author referred to Erickson's office as a "reconverted garage." Further elaboration of this is in Chapter 10 text and Chapter 10, citation 8. (By the way, we really have no idea how far the house was from inside [sic] the garage. We suspect it's much closer than one would think.)
17. Milton Erickson, Ernest Rossi, and Sheila Rossi, *Hypnotic Realities* (New York: Irvington Publishers, 1976), 265.
18. Milton Erickson, *The Collected Papers of Milton H. Erickson, M.D.*, Vol. I, Ernest Rossi, ed. (New York: Irvington Publishers, 1980), 144-145.
19. Milton Erickson, *Healing in Hypnosis*, Ernest Rossi, Margaret Ryan, and Florence Sharp, eds. (New York: Irvington Publishers, 1983), 85.
20. C. Baudoin, *Suggestion et Autosuggestion* (London: George Allen and Unwin, 1921).

Chapter 3

1. Richard Bandler and John Grinder, *The Structure of Magic*, Vol. 1 (Palo Alto, CA: Science and Behavior Books, 1975). In NLP trainings, the Meta Model is generally taught as a systematic way to ask questions which will directionalize the client's experience toward specifics. Modeled primarily from the work of Virginia Satir through the lens of Transformational Grammar, it was designed to assist clients in discovering the deep structure (internal representation) of experience and to fill gaps in their model of the world. It moves the client from an impoverished model of the world to a more detailed and specific model of the world. It is a method of linguistically taking apart a problem. Therefore, the Meta Model is more often used to bring the client out of their "problem trance."

   However, if you focus on one of the Meta Model categories referred to as "deletions," and ask for specifics about a previous trance experience, the more detail that is supplied, the more likely you'll install the state associated with the experience. For a more detailed account of the Meta Model see the Appendix.
2. Richard Bandler and John Grinder, *Frogs Into Princes* (Moab, UT: Real People Press, 1979), 79-136. Anchoring is the term that Bandler and Grinder coined to denote Pavlovian Classical Conditioning. It is the pairing of associations to create a stimulus-response. It is useful in therapy because it enables the therapist to stabilize and activate states with the client. What we refer to as a "naturalistic anchor" in the text is the client's automatic self-talk, auditory analogs, and gestures which are associated with a specific state.
3. Milton Erickson and Herbert Lustig, *The Artistry of Milton H. Erickson* (videotape) (New York: Irvington, 1975). This is a videotape of Dr. Erickson working with a woman named Monde, hence the reference, "The Monde Tapes."
4. John Grinder, Judith DeLozier, and Richard Bandler, *Patterns of the Hypnotic Techniques of Milton H. Erickson, M.D.*, Vol. 2 (Cupertino, CA: Meta Publications, 1977), 140-141. This book contains a verbatim transcript of the Monde tapes which the authors analyzed linguistically.
5. Ibid., 141 and 150.
6. Milton Erickson, "The interpersonal hypnotic technique for symptoms correction and pain control," in *The Collected Papers of Milton H. Erickson, M.D.*, Vol. IV, Ernest Rossi, ed. (New York: Irvington Publishers, 1980), 262-278.
7. Milton Erickson, Ernest Rossi, and Sheila Rossi, *Hypnotic Realities* (New York: Irvington Publishers, 1976), 18.
8. Jay Haley and Madeleine Richeport, *Milton H. Erickson, M.D.: Explorer in Hypnosis and Therapy* (videotape) (New York: Brunner/Mazel, 1993).7. Jeffrey Zeig, *A Teaching Seminar with Milton H. Erickson* (New York: Brunner/Mazel,1980), 63.

9. Milton Erickson and Ernest Rossi, *Hypnotherapy: An Exploratory Casebook* (New York: Irvington Publishers, 1979), 4. Note: This is a recent source and this same concept has been mentioned throughout the literature since James Braid published *Neurypnology: Or the Rationale of Nervous Sleep Considered in Relation to Animal Magnetism* in 1843. In *The Psychology of Suggestion,* published in 1898, Boris Sidis claimed that "the first and general condition of normal suggestibility is fixation of attention."
10. Milton Erickson, Ernest Rossi, and Sheila Rossi, *Hypnotic Realities* (New York: Irvington Publishers, 1976), 21.
11. Stephen and Carol Lankton, *The Answer Within: The Clinical Framework of Ericksonian Hypnotherapy* (New York: Brunner/Mazel, 1983), 247-311.

Chapter 4

1. Milton Erickson, Ernest Rossi, and Sheila Rossi, *Hypnotic Realities* (New York: Irvington Publishers, 1976), 267.
2. Robert Ornstein, *The Psychology of Consciousness,* 2nd Edition (New York: Harcourt Brace Jovanovich, 1977), 37.
3. Michael Talbot, *The Holographic Universe* (New York: HarperCollins, 1991), 17. Talbot refers extensively to the work of Karl Pribram, a Nobel Prize recipient in memory research. Pribram's original work is worth perusing, although it is written in a more academic style than you will find in Talbot's presentation.
4. Deepak Chopra, *Quantum Healing* (New York: Bantam Books, 1989).
5. Candace Pert, "The Chemical Communicators," in Bill Moyers, *Healing and the Mind* (New York: Doubleday, 1993), 193.
6. Richard Bandler and John Grinder, *Frogs Into Princes* (Moab, UT: Real People Press,1979), 160.
7. Leslie LeCron, *Self-Hypnotism* (Englewood Cliffs, NJ: Prentice-Hall, Inc., 1964), 35.
8. J. Allan Hobson, *The Dreaming Brain* (New York: Basic Books, 1988), 295-297.

Chapter 5

1. J. M. Charcot, "Notes sur les divers états nerveux déterminés par l'hypnotization sur les hystéro-épileptiques," presented to the French Academy of Science, February 13, 1882.
2. Milton Erickson, *Mind-Body Communication in Hypnosis,* Ernest Rossi and Margaret Ryan, eds. (New York: Irvington Publishers, 1986), 201-202.
3. William Kroger, *Clinical and Experimental Hypnosis,* 2nd Edition (Philadelphia, PA: J.B. Lippincott Company, 1977), 55.

4. Roger Brown and Richard Hernstein, *Psychology* (Boston, MA: Little, Brown, and Co., 1975), 632.
5. Ernest Rossi, *The Psychobiology of Mind-Body Healing* (New York: W.W. Norton, 1986), 79.
6. Deepak Chopra, *Quantum Healing* (New York: Bantam Books, 1989).
7. Jeffrey Zeig, *A Teaching Seminar with Milton H. Erickson* (New York: Brunner/Mazel, 1980), 63.
8. Milton Erickson, Ernest Rossi, and Sheila Rossi, *Hypnotic Realities* (New York: Irvington Publishers, 1976), 201.
9. Milton Erickson, *Healing in Hypnosis,* Ernest Rossi, Margaret Ryan, and Florence Sharp, eds. (New York: Irvington Publishers, 1983), 110.
10. Georgi Polya, *Patterns of Plausible Inference* (Princeton, NJ: Princeton University Press, 1954).

Chapter 6

1. Submodalities, an area of study within NLP, are the finer distinctions within each external sensory modality, as well as our internal representation of experience. For example, within the visual modality are the submodalities of size, brightness, distance, location, relative motion, focus, etc. These characteristics are one way that our brain makes distinctions. For instance, if you picture someone you like versus someone you dislike, you will probably notice differences in the aforementioned submodalities. In the text, we mentioned that it is possible to elicit the submodalities of an event when an individual experienced time moving slowly and another event when they experienced time moving very quickly. The idea is if we are capable of making distinctions, then the brain must have a way of making those distinctions. Submodalities are NLP's answer to how we encode subjective experience. The original source of submodalities is Richard Bandler, *Using Your Brain for a Change* (Moab, UT: Real People Press, 1985).
2. John Grinder, Judith DeLozier, and Richard Bandler, *Patterns of the Hypnotic Techniques of Milton H. Erickson, M.D.,* Vol. 2 (Cupertino, CA: Meta Publications, 1977), 155-159.
3. John Grinder and Richard Bandler, *TRANCE-formations* (Moab, UT: Real People Press, 1981), 178-184.
4. George Estabrooks, *Hypnotism* (New York: E.P. Dutton, 1943), 192. The concept that the client will tend to actualize what the therapist believes is one of the underlying theses of this book and probably his work in general. In his book he referred to this idea as "operator attitude." If the subject suspects that the operator doubts his success or expects the experiment to be a failure, it will fail. But if the operator is convinced the subject will succeed, then at least in some cases, the subject *will* succeed.
5. Robert Ornstein, *The Psychology of Consciousness,* 2nd Edition (New York: Harcourt Brace Jovanovich, 1977), 52-56.

6. Jay Haley and Madeleine Richeport, *Milton H. Erickson, M.D.: Explorer in Hypnosis and Therapy* (videotape) (New York: Brunner/Mazel, 1993).
7. Milton Erickson, *Healing in Hypnosis*, Ernest Rossi, Margaret Ryan, and Florence Sharp, eds. (New York: Irvington Publishers, 1983), 110. Another important contribution of Erickson's was the idea that pain is a complex. This complex consists of present pain, past pain, and future pain. Past pain refers to sense memories triggered by the present pain which are similar in nature. Future pain is anticipated pain that is related to the expected limitations as a result of the present pain. Clearing the past and future pain will make any intervention on the present pain much easier. *Also see:* Milton Erickson, "An introduction to the study and application of hypnosis for pain control," from *The Collected Papers of Milton H. Erickson, M.D.*, Vol. IV, Ernest Rossi, ed. (New York: Irvington Publishers, 1980), 238.
8. Richard Bandler and John Grinder, *Frogs into Princes* (Moab, UT: Real People Press, 1979), 125. **Note:** We now use the term "V-K Dissociation." At the time of publication John and Richard referred to it as "the two-step visual/kinesthetic dissociation process."
9. Milton Erickson, "Hypnotic Psychotherapy," *The Medical Clinics of North America,* May 1948, New York number, 571-583.
10. Milton Erickson, *Creative Choice,* Ernest Rossi and Margaret Ryan, eds. (New York: Irvington Publishers, 1992), 26.
11. Herbert Spiegel and David Spiegel, *Trance and Treatment: Clinical Uses of Hypnosis* (New York: Basic Books, 1978), 230-232.
12. Tad James and Wyatt Woodsmall, *Time Line Therapy and the Basis of Personality* (Cupertino, CA: Meta Publications, 1988), 36, 38.
13. Boris Sidis, *Psychology of Suggestion* (New York: Appleton & Co., 1898), 71. Sidis has a wonderful quote about dissociation and its relationship to hypnosis and hypnotic phenomena: "Dissociation is the secret of hypnosis and amnesia is the ripe fruit."

Chapter 7

1. Milton Erickson, *Creative Choice in Hypnosis,* Ernest Rossi and Margaret Ryan, eds. (New York: Irvington Publishers, 1992), 5.
2. Jeffrey Zeig, *Experiencing Erickson: An Introduction to the Man and His Work* (New York: Brunner/Mazel, 1985), 38-40. This reference details Zeig's description of Erickson's utilization approach. It gives the reader some insight into what information Erickson thought was useful to elicit from the client.
3. John Grinder, Judith DeLozier, and Richard Bandler, *Patterns of the Hypnotic Techniques of Milton H. Erickson, M.D.*, Vol. 2 (Cupertino, CA: Meta Publications, 1977), 140.
4. Ibid., 143.

5. Milton Erickson, "Pseudo-orientation in time as a therapeutic procedure," *Journal of Clinical and Experimental Hypnosis* 2 (1954): 261-283.
6. Milton Erickson, *Life Reframing in Hypnosis,* Ernest Rossi and Margaret Ryan, eds. (New York: Irvington Publishers, 1985), 200-201.
7. Milton Erickson and Ernest Rossi, *Hypnotherapy: An Exploratory Casebook* (New York: Irvington Publishers, 1979), 103-104.
8. Milton Erickson, *Mind-Body Communication in Hypnosis,* Ernest Rossi and Margaret Ryan, eds. (New York: Irvington Publishers, 1986), 248. In reference to Erickson's use of reframing in mind-body problems, Rossi concludes, "The key to mind-body communication and healing is to access and reframe the state-dependent memory and learning systems that encode symptoms and life problems."
9. Milton Erickson and Ernest Rossi, *Hypnotherapy: An Exploratory Casebook* (New York: Irvington Publishers, 1979), 102-122.
10. Milton Erickson, "Varieties of hypnotic amnesia," *The Collected Papers of Milton H. Erickson, M.D.,* Vol. III, Ernest Rossi, ed. (New York: Irvington Publishers, 1980), 90. Erickson summarized this point by saying, "Hypnotic amnesia is thus a convenient approach for coping with consciousness and protecting therapeutic suggestions from the limitations of the patient's conscious mental sets."
11. Milton Erickson, *Healing in Hypnosis,* Ernest Rossi, Margaret Ryan, and Florence Sharp, eds. (New York: Irvington Publishers, 1983), 6.
12. Sidney Rosen, ed., *My Voice Will Go with You* (New York: W.W. Norton, 1982), 108-109.

Chapter 8

1. Milton Erickson and Elizabeth Erickson, "Concerning the nature and character of posthypnotic behavior," in *The Collected Papers of Milton H. Erickson,* Vol. I, Ernest Rossi, ed. (New York: Irvington Publishers, 1980), 381-411.
2. George Estabrooks, *Hypnotism* (New York: Dutton & Co.,1943), 70.
3. Andre Weitzenhoffer, *The Practice of Hypnotism,* Vol. 1 (New York: John Wiley & Sons, 1989), 258.
4. Ibid., 260.
5. Milton Erickson and Elizabeth Erickson, "Concerning the nature and character of post-hypnotic behavior," in *The Collected Papers of Milton H. Erickson,* Vol. I , Ernest Rossi, ed. (New York: Irvington Publishers, 1980), 381-411.
6. E. Gurney, "Peculiarities of certain posthypnotic states," *Proceedings of the Society for Psychic Research* 4, 1886, 268-323.
7. William Kroger, *Clinical and Experimental Hypnosis,* 2nd Edition (Philadelphia, PA: J. B. Lippincott Co., 1977), 14.

8. William James, *Principles of Psychology* (Chicago: William Benton, 1952), 841-842. This psychology textbook, which can be found in the original two-volume set or the abridged version, devotes an entire chapter to hypnotism, along with an excellent chapter on "imagination" in which he discusses ideas that later show up in modern neuro-linguistics.
9. Stephen and Carol Lankton, *The Answer Within: A Clinical Framework of Ericksonian Hypnotherapy* (New York: Brunner/Mazel, 1983), 247-311.
10. Milton Erickson and Elizabeth Erickson, "Concerning the nature and character of posthypnotic behavior," in *The Collected Papers of Milton H. Erickson,* Vol. I, Ernest Rossi, ed., (New York: Irvington Publishers, 1980), 381-411.
11. John Grinder and Richard Bandler, *TRANCE-formations* (Moab, UT: Real People Press, 1981), 70-77.

Chapter 9

1. Gregory Bateson and Mary Bateson, *Angels Fear: Towards an Epistemology of the Sacred* (New York: Macmillan, 1987).
2. A. B. Lord, *The Singer of Tales* (Cambridge, MA: Harvard University Press, 1960).
3. W. J. Ong, *Orality and Literacy: The Technologizing of the Word* (London: Methuen, 1982).
4. W. J. Ong, *Interfaces of the Word: Studies in the Evolution of Consciousness and Culture* (Ithaca, NY: Cornell University Press, 1977), 69.
5. Ibid, 69.
6. David Gordon, *Therapeutic Metaphors* (Cupertino, CA: Meta Publications, 1978), 40.
7. Alfred Korzybski, *Science and Sanity* (Lakeville, CT: The International Non-Aristotelian Library Publishing Company, 1933), 63. **Note:** Korzybski's exact quote, from which we have inferred that, "all meaning is context dependent" is: "More than that, as the only possible content of knowledge and science is structural, whether we like it or not, to *know* anything we must search for structure, or posit some structure." (Emphasis is Korzybski's.)
8. Stephen Lankton, *Ericksonian Therapy* (Cape Cod Symposium: August 19-23, 1991), audiotapes 1-10.
9. I. Yaniv and D. E. Meyer, "Activation and metacognition of inaccessible stored information: Potential bases for incubation effects in problem solving," *Journal of Experimental Psychology: Learning, Memory, and Cognition* 13, 187-205.
10. S. M. Kosslyn, "The medium and the message in mental imagery: A theory," *Psychological Review* 88, 46-66.
11. A. Rothenberg, *The Creative Process of Psychotherapy* (New York: W. W. Norton, 1988).

12. Edward DeBono, *New Think* (New York: Avon Books, 1967), 17-27.
13. Stephen and Carol Lankton, *The Answer Within: The Clinical Framework of Ericksonian Hypnotherapy* (New York: Brunner/Mazel, 1983).
14. W. J. Ong, *Orality and Literacy: The Technologizing of the Word* (London, Methuen, 1982), 27.
15. H. Ebbinghaus, *Memory: A Contribution to Experimental Psychology* (New York: Teacher's College, Columbia University, 1913).
16. S. Sternberg, "Memory scanning: New findings and current controversies," *Quarterly Journal of Experimental Psychology* 22 (1975): 1-32.
17. Gregory Bateson and Mary Bateson, *Angels Fear: Towards an Epistemology of the Sacred* (New York: Macmillan, 1987), 13.
18. Ibid.
19. Ibid., 10.
20. Peter Brown, *The Hypnotic Brain* (New Haven, CT: Yale University Press, 1991), 79.

Chapter 10

1. Milton Erickson, *Life Reframing in Hypnosis,* Ernest Rossi and Margaret Ryan, eds. (New York: Irvington Publishers, 1985).
2. Jeffrey Zeig, *A Teaching Seminar with Milton H. Erickson* (New York: Brunner/Mazel, 1980).
3. Milton Erickson and Ernest Rossi, *Hypnotherapy: An Exploratory Casebook* (New York: Irvington Publishers, 1979).
4. Milton Erickson, "Hypnosis in medical practice: three case histories," in *The Collected Papers of Milton H. Erickson,* Vol. IV, Ernest Rossi, ed. (New York: Irvington Publishers, 1980), 58-66.
5. Stephen Gilligan, *Therapeutic Trances* (New York: Brunner/Mazel, 1987), 314.
6. Andre Weitzenhoffer, *The Practice of Hypnotism,* Vol. 2 (New York: John Wiley & Sons, Inc., 1989), 130-132.
7. Swami Shri Kripalvanandji, *Premyatra: Pilgrimage of Love,* Book 1 (Lenox, MA: Kripalu Yoga Fellowship, 1992), 69-70.
8. Stephen Lankton, *Ericksonian Therapy* (Cape Cod Symposium: August 19-23, 1991), audiotapes 1-10. **Note:** In these tapes we recall the author referring to Erickson's office as a "reconverted garage." If it's not there then, "Thank you, Steve" for stimulating this association for us. In *Healing and Hypnosis* and in *A Teaching Seminar with Milton H. Erickson,* references are made to his office as a guesthouse. Our preference for the garage, rather than the guesthouse, is based upon all the associations which the former naturally engenders.

9. Milton Erickson, "Hypnosis in medical practice: three case histories," in *The Collected Papers of Milton H. Erickson,* Vol. IV, Ernest Rossi, ed. (New York: Irvington Publishers, 1980), 58-66.
10. Stephen Gilligan, *Therapeutic Trances* (New York: Brunner/Mazel, 1987), 314.
11. John Grinder, Judith DeLozier, and Richard Bandler, *Patterns of the Hypnotic Techniques of Milton H. Erickson, M.D.,* Vol. 2 (Cupertino, CA: Meta Publications, 1977), 155.
12. Milton Erickson, *Life Reframing in Hypnosis,* Ernest Rossi and Margaret Ryan, eds. (New York: Irvington Publishers, 1985), 225-226.
13. Milton Erickson, *Life Reframing in Hypnosis,* Ernest Rossi and Margaret Ryan, eds. (New York: Irvington Publishers, 1985), 225.
14. Stephen LaBerge, *Lucid Dreaming* (New York: Ballantine Books, 1985), 171.

Appendix

Note To The Reader:

The contents of the Appendix, with the exception of "Installation of Peripheral Vision," are excerpts from our NLP Practitioner Training Manual. We decided to keep the contents in "bullet" form, as they appear in the manual, to highlight only the important points of each subject area.

1. Facilitating Peripheral Vision
2. Milton Model
3. Meta Model
4. Visual-Kinesthetic Dissociation
5. The Conditions of A Well-Formed Outcome
6. Reframing

---

1. FACILITATING PERIPHERAL VISION

"If you would, just go ahead and find a point out in front of you and slightly above eye level . . . Now . . . fix your gaze on that point and keep it there . . . notice whatever details you can about the point . . . As you keep your eyes fixed on that point you may begin to become aware of the front corners of the room . . . (Begin to mention any other objects that the client may see that would be to the right and left of the original point and begin expanding their distance all the way to the front sides of the room.) *That's right . . . just allow your awareness to expand . . . not only your visual awareness, but you might also notice how your hearing and feeling may be expanding into the same space as well . . . Now continue expanding your awareness all the way out to the sides of the room . . . "*

OPTIONAL: (Begin to wave your hand about two feet from the side of the client's head.) . . . *You may even begin to notice my hand here on the periphery* . . . (wait until client acknowledges this) . . . *and continue if you will to **expand your awareness** to the space behind you . . . that's right . . . this is **peripheral vision**"* (mark this out analogically within your voice).

At this point, the therapist ought to be noticing a number of physiological indications that the client is, indeed, in peripheral vision and parasympathetic arousal (relaxation response). You will usually notice a defocusing of the eyes and a loosening of the muscles around the eyes followed by a concomitant flaccidity of the facial muscles. Observe carefully that the temporomandibular joint (TMJ) is loose. Loosening of the TMJ is often a result of accessing peripheral vision. If you see tightness in this area, suggest relaxation of the jaw. This is important because there is some indication, based on early research in behaviorism, that tension in this area may be accompanied by "subvocal speech" or internal dialogue. Relaxation of the jaw in concert with or as a result of peripheral vision will often interrupt, if not completely silence, internal dialogue. This is a mystical state to which many esoteric traditions refer. Loosening of the facial muscles is usually followed by a noticeable breathing shift—usually lower and deeper in the diaphragm. There are other physiological cues to which one could attend; however, those just mentioned are fairly universal and reliable.

2. THE MILTON MODEL
The Hypnotic Language Patterns of Milton H. Erickson, M.D.

The Milton Model is the inverse of the Meta Model. It creates "artfully vague" language that is ambiguous and abstract. This use of language results in the listener having to perform a transderivational search (TDS) in an attempt to assign meaning to what was said. The listener will unknowingly begin to associate his/her experiences to what was said while, at the same time, accepting the direction and/or boundaries of the speaker. This trance state is known in NLP as "downtime."

Mind Read
"*I know that you are learning . . .*"
Claiming to know the internal process (thoughts and feelings) of another without identifying the process or sensory-based data which was used to determine the information.

Lost Performative
"*And it's a good thing to learn . . .*"
Value judgments where the performer of the judgment has been deleted.

Cause-Effect
"Because..."
Where it is implied or directly stated that one thing causes another. Linguistic markers include: *"makes," "If...then," "As...then."*

Complex Equivalence
"That means..."
Where things—or their meanings—are equated as synonomous.

Presupposition
"You have many valuable skills and resources available to you at a moment's notice..."
The linguistic equivalent of assumptions.

Universal Quantifier
"All the resources you ever needed..."
Words that are absolute generalizations lacking a referential index, such as: *any, always, never, every, all, none,* etc.

Modal Operator
"That you can learn to use..."
Words which dictate or imply what is possible and/or necessary in life.

Nominalization
"In various creative combinations to produce new understandings and abilities that can stay with you the rest of your life..."
A process (stated as a verb) which has been changed to an event (noun).

Unspecified Verb
"And you can..."
Process words which lack a complete description—all verbs are to a greater or lesser degree unspecified.

Tag Question
"Haven't you?..."
A question added at the end of a statement to displace resistance. It will usually create an affirmative answer and can also be accompanied by a temporal shift.

Lack of Referential Index
"And one can, you know . . ."
A phrase which deletes who is doing the acting.

Comparative Deletion
"At the very least, understand even more deeply . . ."
Words which imply a comparison but lack the object on which the comparison is based.

Pace Current Experience
"As you are sitting here, looking at this page and reading this . . ."
Truisms about the listener's current, on-going sensory experience.

Double Bind
"With your conscious mind, while your unconscious mind is learning something else and I don't know whether you'll discover just what you've learned . . . now, in a few moments from now, or sometime later..."
Statements or questions which engage one's attention on a consequence which presupposes something else. It creates what Erickson called "an illusion of choice."

Conversational Postulate
"But could you just look up for a moment?"
A yes/no question to which the listener will respond by actually doing what is implied.

Extended Quote
". . . And looking up reminds me of the time I was instructed to look up as a way to dissociate from unwanted feelings while at a Tony Robbins' firewalk, right before he was telling us about a training he did with John Grinder where John said about ten years ago he was with Richard who once asked someone . . ."
Linguistically chaining a series of contexts which tend to overload one's conscious attention and dissociate what is being said by the speaker.

Ambiguity
- **Phonological**
  "Are you here (pointing to his ear) . . ."
  Homonyms which tend to create mild confusion.

- **Punctuational**
  "What I'm saying . . . just become aware of your head right into trance now . . ."
  Connecting two phrases with one word (e.g. "head") at the end of the first statement and with the first word of the second phrase.

- **Syntactic**
  "Because Training Trances promote healing feelings . . ."
  Where the function of a word cannot be quickly known from the immediate context.

- **Scope**
  " . . . And speaking to you as a healing master, you must realize that by now . . ."
  Where the scope of the linguistic context cannot be determined.

© *1990 Neuro-Energetics*

---

3. THE META MODEL

The Meta Model is a systematic way to increase choice in people's lives. Each person experiences "reality" and codes it with the use of language. Language exists on two levels: Deep Structure—the full linguistic representation of the experience within the person; and Surface Structure—the way a person represents the experience to others. If the surface structure and deep structure match they are said to be "synonymous"; if they do not match, they are "ambiguous." The purpose of the Meta Model is to retrieve information from the source of the ambiguity so that the Surface Structure and Deep Structure match one another.

DISTORTIONS

Cause-Effect
"You make me feel like I'm not perfect."
Where cause for one's behavior or feelings is wrongly attributed to someone or something rather than to oneself.
Metaquestion: How does what _____ is doing cause you to choose to _____?
Metaeffect: Recovers choice.

Complex Equivalence
"When you turn away, you don't think I'm good enough for you."
Two experiences are interpreted as being synonymous when they may not be. When a behavior, etc., is said to mean _____.
Metaquestion: How does his _____ mean he_____? Have you ever _____ someone who you did think was _____?
Metaeffect: Provides counterexample and recovers deep structure complex equivalence.

Mind Read
"He doesn't think I'm good enough."
Claiming to know someone else's internal process (thoughts and feelings) without identifying the process or sensory-based data that was used to determine the information.
Metaquestion: How do you know_____?
Metaeffect: Recovers source of information.

Lost Performative
"You're not good enough unless you're perfect."
Making a value judgment without stating whose opinion it is and acting as if the statement is true.
Metaquestion: Who says _____? According to whom? How do you know it's _____?
Metaeffect: Recovers source of belief, belief strategy.

GENERALIZATIONS

Modal Operators
a. **Modal Operators of Necessity**—verbs which presuppose a need or requirement (should, must, got to, have to, need to, shouldn't, must not). *"I must succeed."*
   Metaquestion: What would happen if you did? What wouldn't happen if you didn't?
   Metaeffect: Recovers effects and outcomes.

b. **Modal Operators of Possibility**—verbs which presuppose choice or possibility (can/can't, will/won't, may/may not, possible/impossible). *"I can't stay in a relationship."*
   Metaquestion: What prevents you? What would happen if you did?
   Metaeffect: Recovers cause.

Universal Quantifiers
"I never do it right."
Nouns, adjectives, or adverbs which presuppose total inclusion or exclusion (all, every, everyone, nobody, never, etc.).
Metaquestion: Never?.All? What would happen if you did? (find counterexample)
Metaeffect: Recover outcome, effects, and counterexample.

DELETIONS

Nominalizations
"My decision created a limitation in my life."
Verbs which are process words but have been turned into nouns, resulting in a static condition.
Metaquestion: How are you deciding to limit yourself now? What unlimited possibilities do you want to be deciding upon now?
Metaeffect: Recovers process.

Unspecified Verbs
"I can't learn."
Verbs which delete information about the process.
Metaquestion: How, specifically _____?
Metaeffect: Recovers process information.

Simple Deletions
a. **Simple deletions** *"I'm not sure."*
   Metaquestion: About what, whom?
   Metaeffect: Recovers deletion.

b. **Lack of referential index—deletes the specific person or thing**
   "They aren't sure."
   Metaquestion: Who, specifically?
   Metaeffect: Recovers referential index.

c. **Comparative deletions**
   "She's more sure."
   Making a comparison without stating what or who's being compared.
   Metaquestion: Compared to whom or what?
   Metaeffect: Recovers comparative deletion.

© 1990 Neuro-Energetics

4. VISUAL-KINESTHETIC DISSOCIATION

This protocol can be used when dealing with overpowering negative kinesthetic responses such as phobias and trauma. The following outline assumes that a congruent outcome has been elicited and a baseline of the problem BMIR (Behavioral Manifestation of Internal Representation) has been calibrated. In cases of phobias and/or extreme trauma, it may be counterproductive to ask the client to associate with the experience (an abreaction may occur). In these cases, calibrate to the problem BMIR while client discusses the problem conversationally.

1. Establish a security **anchor** (also a bailout procedure).
   Calibrate to security BMIR.

2. Have the client see the younger self just before the negative experience in the first frame of a movie which is on a screen far in front and down below them. **Anchor.** (This is the first level of dissociation.)
   Calibrate.

3. Have client float up and out of body. **Anchor.** (This is the second level of dissociation—or double dissociation.)
   Calibrate.

4. Have client watch the movie of their younger self going through the negative experience until the younger self reaches a safe place—or after the trauma has ended. Have client freeze that frame.

5. Have client float back down into their body, **releasing** the double dissociation **anchor.** Calibrate to integration.

6. Have client walk up to younger self on the screen (**release** the dissociation **anchor**) and ask them to comfort their younger self. This is an opportunity for lots of indirect and direct suggestions for acceptance, comfort, learning, security, etc. Be sure to use pace-and-lead statements while watching BMIR for feedback.

7. Have client reintegrate younger self with present self.

8. Reorient to present context.

© 1990 Neuro-Energetics

5. THE CONDITIONS OF A WELL-FORMED OUTCOME

1. Stated in positives—is described in terms of what is wanted, not what isn't wanted.

2. Sensory-based—can be seen, heard, felt, tasted, smelled, etc.

3. Initiated and maintained by individual—the desired state is under control of the individual and is not dependent on someone else or something else.

4. Ecological—fits with the person's personality, family system, overall values, and goals.

5. Preserves positive by-product of present state—adds to the existing choices, rather than eliminating aspects of present state that may be useful.

6. Specific and contextualized—identifies when and how the desired state is wanted.

7. Includes internal process, internal state, external behavior—imagery, cognitions, submodalities, strategies, and behavior.

© *1990 Neuro-Energetics*

6. REFRAMING

Reframing is based on the presupposition that every experience in the world and every behavior is appropriate given some context, some frame.

Reframing changes the individual's internal context.

The behaviors which are most difficult to work with occur when the majority of the client's context is internal.

Two types of reframing:

1. Context—tip-off: "too" much of something
   "I'm too" or "he's too" (comparative generalization)
   To reframe, hold behavior constant and change context: use lead system to assist client in changing contexts.

   "In what context would this particular behavior (that the person is complaining of) have value?"

2. Meaning—tip-off: x causes y (cause-effect)
   $x = y$ (complex equivalence)
   To reframe, hold context constant and change meaning of behavior.

   "Is there a larger or different frame in which this behavior would have a positive value?"

*To execute either type: pace—calibrate—and then lead with the reframe.

© 1990 Neuro-Energetics

Bibliography

Baars, B. J. *A Cognitive Theory of Consciousness*. Cambridge: Cambridge University Press, 1988.

Bandler, Richard. *Time For A Change*. Cupertino, CA: Meta Publications, 1993.

Bandler, Richard and John Grinder. *Frogs Into Princes*. Moab, UT: Real People Press, 1979.

———. *The Structure of Magic*, Vol. I. Palo Alto, CA: Science and Behavior Books, 1975.

———. *Patterns of the Hypnotic Techniques of Milton H. Erickson, M.D.*, Vol. I. Cupertino, CA: Meta Publications, 1977.

———. *Reframing*. Moab, UT: Real People Press, 1982.

Barber, Joseph and Cheri Adrian, eds. *Psychological Approaches to the Management of Pain*. New York: Brunner/Mazel, 1982.

Bateson, Gregory and Mary Bateson. *Angels Fear: Towards an Epistemology of the Sacred*. New York: Macmillan, 1987.

Baudoin, C. *Suggestion et Autosuggestion*. London: George Allen and Unwin, 1921.

Brown, Peter. *The Hypnotic Brain*. New Haven, CT: Yale University Press, 1991.

Brown, Roger and Richard Hernstein. *Psychology*. Boston, MA: Little, Brown and Co., 1975.

Chopra, Deepak. *Quantum Healing*. New York: Bantam Books, 1989.

DeBono, Edward. *New Think*. New York: Avon Books, 1967.

Ebbinghaus, H. *Memory: A Contribution to Experimental Psychology*. New York: Teacher's College, Columbia University, 1913.

Erickson, Milton. *The Collected Papers of Milton H. Erickson,* Vol. I, edited by Ernest Rossi. New York: Irvington Publishers, 1980.

_____. *The Collected Papers of Milton H. Erickson*, Vol. II, edited by Ernest Rossi. New York: Irvington Publishers, 1980.

_____. *The Collected Papers of Milton H. Erickson*, Vol. III, edited by Ernest Rossi. New York: Irvington Publishers, 1980.

_____. *The Collected Papers of Milton H. Erickson*, Vol. IV, edited by Ernest Rossi. New York: Irvington Publishers, 1980.

Erickson, Milton, Seymour Hershman, and Irving Secter. *The Practical Application of Medical and Dental Hypnosis*. New York: Brunner/Mazel, 1961.

Erickson, Milton. *Healing in Hypnosis*, edited by Ernest Rossi, Margaret Ryan, and Florence Sharp. New York: Irvington Publishers, 1983.

Erickson, Milton and Ernest Rossi. *Hypnotherapy: An Exploratory Casebook*. New York: Irvington Publishers, 1976.

Erickson, Milton, Ernest Rossi and Sheila Rossi. *Hypnotic Realities*. New York: Irvington Publishers, 1976.

Erickson, Milton. *Life Reframing in Hypnosis*, edited by Ernest Rossi and Margaret Ryan. New York: Irvington Publishers, 1985.

Erickson, Milton. *Mind-Body Communication in Hypnosis*, edited by Ernest Rossi and Margaret Ryan. New York: Irvington Publishers, 1985.

_____. *Creative Choice in Hypnosis*, edited by Ernest Rossi and Margaret Ryan. New York: Irvington Publishers, 1992.

Estabrooks, George. *Hypnotism*. New York: E. P. Dutton, 1943.

Gackenbach, Jayne and Jane Bosweld. *Control Your Dreams*. New York: Harper Perennial, 1989.

Garfield, Patricia. *Creative Dreaming*. New York: Ballantine Books, 1974.

Gilligan, Stephen. *Therapeutic Trances*. New York: Brunner/Mazel, 1987.

Gordon, David. *Therapeutic Metaphors*. Cupertino, CA: Meta Publications, 1978.

Gordon, David and Maribeth Meyers-Anderson. *Phoenix: Therapeutic Patterns of Milton H. Erickson*. Cupertino, CA: Meta Publications, 1981.

Grinder, John and Richard Bandler. *The Structure of Magic*, Vol. II. Palo Alto, CA: Science and Behavior Books, 1976.

_____. *TRANCE-formations*. Moab, UT: Real People Press, 1981.

_____. *Patterns of the Hypnotic Techniques of Milton H. Erickson, M.D.*, Vol. II. Cupertino, CA: Meta Publications, 1977.

Haley, Jay. *Advanced Techniques of Hypnosis and Therapy: Selected Papers of Milton H. Erickson, M.D.* New York: Grune and Stratton, 1967.

Hobson, J. Alan. *The Dreaming Brain: How the Brain Creates Both the Sense and the Nonsense of Dreams.* New York: Basic Books, 1988.

Hulse, Stewart, James Deese, and Howard Egeth. *The Psychology of Learning,* 4th Edition. New York: McGraw-Hill, 1975.

James, Tad and Wyatt Woodsmall. *Time Line Therapy and the Basis of Personality.* Cupertino, CA: Meta Publications, 1988.

James, William. *The Principles of Psychology.* Chicago, IL: William Benton, 1952.

Korzybski, Alfred. *Science and Sanity,* 4th Edition. Lakeville, CT: The International Non-Aristotelian Library Publishing Co., 1933.

Kripalvanandji, Swami Shri. *Premyatra: Pilgrimage of Love,* Book 1. Lenox, MA: Kripalu Yoga Fellowship, 1992.

Kroger, William. *Clinical and Experimental Hypnosis,* 2nd Edition. Philadelphia, PA: J. B. Lippincott Company, 1977.

Lankton, Stephen and Carol Lankton. *The Answer Within: A Clinical Framework of Ericksonian Hypnotherapy.* New York: Brunner/Mazel, 1983.

LaBerge, Stephen. *Lucid Dreaming.* New York: Ballantine Books, 1985.

LeCron, Leslie. *Self-Hypnotism.* Englewood Cliffs, NJ: Prentice-Hall, 1964.

Lewicki, P. *Nonconscious Social Information Processing.* Orlando, FL: Academic Press, 1986.

Lewis, Byron and R. Frank Pucelik. *Magic Demystified.* Portland, OR: Metamorphous Press, 1982.

Lord, A. B. *The Singer of Tales.* Cambridge, MA: Harvard University Press, 1980.

Moyers, Bill. *Healing and the Mind.* New York: Doubleday, 1993.

O'Hanlon, William Hudson and Angela Hexum. *An Uncommon Casebook: The Complete Clinical Work of Milton H. Erickson, M.D.* New York: W. W. Norton, 1990.

Ong, W. J. *Interfaces of the Word: Studies in the Evolution of Consciousness and Culture.* Ithaca, NY: Cornell University, 1977.

———. *Orality and Literacy: The Technologizing of the Word.* London: Methuen, 1982.

Ornstein, Robert. *The Psychology of Consciousness,* 2nd Edition. New York: Harcourt Brace Jovanovich, 1977.

Ostrander, Sheila, Lynn Schroeder, and Nancy Ostrander. *Superlearning.* New York: Laurel, 1979.

Penfield, Wilder. *The Mystery of the Mind: A Critical Study of Consciousness and the Human Brain.* Princeton, NJ: Princeton University Press, 1975.

Polya, Georgi. *Patterns of Plausible Inference.* Princeton, NJ: Princeton Press, 1954.

Pribram, Karl. *Languages of the Brain,* 5th Edition. Monterey, CA: Wadsworth Publishing, 1977.

Rosen, Sidney, ed. *My Voice Will Go With You.* New York: W. W. Norton, 1982.

Rossi, Ernest. *The Psychobiology of Mind-Body Healing.* New York: W. W. Norton, 1986.

Rothenberg, A. *The Creative Process of Psychotherapy.* New York: W. W. Norton, 1988.

Sidis, Boris. *Psychology of Suggestion.* New York: Appleton & Co., 1898.

Spiegel, Herbert and David Spiegel. *Trance and Treatment: Clinical Uses of Hypnosis.* New York: Basic Books, 1978.

Talbot, Michael. *The Holographic Universe.* New York: HarperCollins, 1991.

Weitzenhoffer, Andre. *The Practice of Hypnotism,* Vol. 1. New York: John Wiley & Sons, 1989.

_____. *The Practice of Hypnotism,* Vol. 2. New York: John Wiley & Sons, 1989.

Wolf, Fred Alan. *The Dreaming Universe.* New York: Simon & Schuster, 1994.

Zeig, Jeffrey. *A Teaching Seminar with Milton H. Erickson.* New York: Brunner/Mazel, 1980.

_____. *Experiencing Erickson: An Introduction to the Man and His Work.* New York: Brunner/Mazel, 1985.

Index

age regression
 103, 110, 119, 207
agonist muscles
 47, 82, 96
alignment
 5, 141, 150, 158
altered state 7, 11
ambiguous touch 90
amnesia
 8, 21, 97, 103, 106,
 110, 116, 123, 124,
 130, 131, 142, 143,
 144, 149, 151, 155,
 156, 157, 159, 160,
 161, 174, 181, 193,
 201, 207, 212
analgesia
 82, 97, 101, 103,
 107, 110, 111, 112,
 113, 114, 117, 123,
 124, 207
glove analgesia 97
analog 135, 171, 192
analog, voice
 41, 44, 185
analogs, trance 44
anchor
 42, 44, 183, 185,
 191, 192, 196, 223
anesthesia
 82, 107, 111, 117,
 124
antagonist muscles
 47, 82, 96, 105
apposition of opposites
 99
archetype 130
arm catalepsy
 47, 83, 92, 97, 111
arm levitation
 82, 83, 99, 105

association
 12, 20, 104, 117
associations 167, 201
autonomic nervous
 system 3, 5
autosuggestion 149

balanced tonicity 105
Bandler, Richard 9, 161
Bateson, Gregory
 165, 181
BMIR 223
bodymind 104
boundary condition
 118, 135
breathing 57, 67
Buddhism 119
bushy-brained 165, 171

**calibration
 9, 11, 17, 20,**
 43, 58, 167, 173,
 185, 223, 225
catalepsy
 35, 47, 79, 81, 82,
 83, 85, 86, 87, 90,
 91, 94, 96, 97, 98,
 99, 100, 101, 104,
 105, 108, 110, 113,
 117, 121, 122, 124,
 134, 144, 192, 198,
 200
catatonia 82, 105
cause-effect 218, 220
changework
 18, 38, 42, 128,
 131, 135, 136, 140,
 142, 146, 156, 158,
 159
Charcot, J. M. 81
Christianity 119
chunking down
 42, 43, 44, 129, 130

chunking up
 69, 136, 172
comparative deletion
 219, 222
complex equivalence
 218, 221
congruency
 17, 89, 131, 136, 158
Conscious-Unconscious
 Dissociation 2, 41, 60,
 61, 62, 67, 68, 70, 71,
 74, 75, 82, 89, 97,
 116, 117, 128, 132,
 133, 134, 144, 146,
 158, 159, 160, 161,
 185, 192, 196
consciousness 2
content
 129, 132, 133, 143,
 161, 168
context
 3, 43, 136, 138, 140,
 150, 168
conversational postulate
 219
convincer 77, 103
cortical stimulation 7
creativity
 62, 166, 171, 201
Cybervision 119

DeBono, Edward 172
Deep Trance
 Identification (DTI)
 97, 103, 109, 110,
 117, 118, 119, 120,
 121, 122
deletions 222
dental pain 100
direct suggestion
 15, 18, 19, 20, 21,
 103, 113
disorientation 150

Index   233

disorientation of body 108
disorientation of space 108
disorientation of time 107
dissociation
   62, 67, 97, 100, 107, 114, 131, 185, 196
distortion 220
distraction
   112, 113, 128, 143, 146, 162
double bind
   77, 169, 171, 219
double dissociation 223
double induction
   15, 23, 161
downtime 12, 217
downtime trance 36, 38
dream
   6, 20, 37, 79, 84, 107, 116, 123, 141, 155, 198, 199, 201
lucid dream 201
dream state 7
driving trance
   15, 23, 32, 204

ecology
   59, 106, 109, 114, 115, 118, 121, 122, 124, 131, 181, 224
embedded commands
   47, 51, 130, 155
embedded suggestions 103
Erickson, Milton
   1, 2, 3, 4, 6, 7, 8, 9, 10, 15, 17, 19, 21, 22, 25, 31, 35, 36, 41, 42, 43, 44, 47, 50, 51, 52, 61, 67, 68, 69, 81, 85, 90, 91, 95, 99, 100, 106, 107, 110, 112, 114, 115, 124, 125, 127,

129, 130, 134, 135, 140, 143, 144, 147, 149, 150, 151, 155, 156, 157, 165, 166, 167, 168, 183, 185, 189, 192, 193, 194, 200, 217, 219
Estabrooks, George
   16, 110, 149
extended quote 219
eyeblink reflex
   53, 67, 92, 94

fixation 51, 100, 162
fixation of attention
   71, 183
fractionation
   47, 155, 200
Freud, Sigmund 4
future pace 142, 154

generalizations 221
generative work 158
Gilligan, Stephen 194
Grinder, John 219
Gurney, E. 150

habituation 112
Haley, Jay 10
hallucination 103
handshake induction
   83, 85, 90, 161
Hawaiian healers 168
healing
   82, 100, 101, 102, 104, 114, 118, 153, 160
hemispheres, brain
   51, 62
Hinduism 119
holographic model
   3, 62, 103
Hull, Clark 16
hypnogogic 7, 201
hypnopompic 7, 201
hypnosis, traditional
   16, 21, 98, 103, 157, 184

hypnotic dream induction
   183, 194, 200, 201, 202
hypnotic interview
   41, 127, 128, 131, 143, 146, 159, 196
hypnotic phenomena
   60, 81, 97, 103, 104, 111, 122, 128, 134, 140, 141, 144, 146, 152, 156, 158, 159, 166, 185

ideomotor signals
   60, 61, 68, 70, 73, 75, 77, 82, 110, 134, 135
incongruency 17
indirect suggestion
   15, 18, 19, 21, 68, 77, 103, 128, 139, 144, 155, 157, 159
induction 173
intake process 129
internal representation 72
interspersal technique 47
involuntary functions 101
IPA 5
isomorphism 168

kinesthetic ambiguity 86, 89

lack of referential index
   219, 222
Lankton, Stephen
   155, 168, 173, 180
latent learning 5
law of reverse effect 38
layering 55, 161, 173
leading
   53, 67, 111, 113, 120, 122, 159, 192, 223
learning to learn 181
LeCron, Leslie 69
Libet, Benjamin 3, 5

linguistic markers 117
loops 15, 156, 165, 183
  nested 59, 155, 173
  open 156, 174
  sub-loop 180
lost performative
  217, 221

Master Woodcutter
  165, 174, 202
matching
  17, 35, 43, 45, 49,
  53, 60, 67, 79,
  95, 173
memories 141
Meta Model
  42, 43, 49, 216,
  217, 220
meta-outcome 103, 183
metaphor 2, 165
  boat metaphor 186
  construction 166
  garage metaphor
    26, 193
  Kleenex metaphor 169
  mango metaphor
    188, 191
  meal metaphor 153
  mirror metaphor 115
  perfect circle metaphor
    186
  theater metaphor 115
  therapeutic 16
  tiger metaphor 112
Metaphorical
  Intervention
  183, 185, 192, 196,
  202
metaprogram 181
method acting 110, 118
micro movements 119
Milton Model
  19, 42, 98, 216, 217
mind read
  136, 137, 217, 221
mirroring
  17, 35, 43, 45, 49,
  53, 60, 67, 79, 173
mismatch 96

mnemonics 167
modal operator 218
modal operator of
  necessity 221
model operator of
  possibility 221
Monde Tape
  44, 107, 130
multi-embedded metaphor
  59, 155, 173, 174

negative hallucination
  109, 112, 119
neural networks
  68, 129, 135, 137,
  141, 185
neural transmission 118
neuropeptides 3
new behavior 149, 155
New Behavior Generator
  110
Neurolinguistic
  Programming (NLP)
  1, 9, 39, 42, 44, 76,
  110, 114, 115, 129,
  131, 135, 151, 154,
  160, 162, 165, 169,
  184, 194, 217
nominalization
  2, 218, 222
nonverbal suggestion 85

Ong, W. J. 167, 173
oral poets 167
oral tradition 166
ordeals 8, 169, 171
outcome state 129, 137
overload
  85, 160, 161, 174,
  219
overwhelm 168

pacing
  17, 53, 82, 90, 95,
  96, 97, 111, 113, 117,
  120, 122, 129, 159,
  185, 192, 223, 225

Pacing Current
  Experience
  41, 51, 52, 54, 55,
  58, 59, 60, 65, 67,
  156, 219
pain
  100, 104, 106, 112,
  114, 115, 124, 138,
  162
parallel construction
  57, 59
parallel layering 174
parallel processing 6
part 118
pattern interrupt
  85, 86, 90, 150
peripheral vision
  216, 217
permissive approach 16
phantom pain 140, 141
phantom pleasure 140
phobias 223
Phoenix 147
phonological ambiguity
  219
plausibility 101
positive hallucination
  103, 108, 109, 138,
  140
positive internal
  representation
  38, 39, 157
posthypnotic behavior
  149, 150, 151, 154,
  157
posthypnotic suggestion
  49, 54, 57, 58, 75,
  97, 111, 122, 128,
  141, 144, 146, 149,
  150, 151, 152, 154,
  155, 157, 158, 159,
  162, 163, 184, 185,
  193
preframe 94, 174
premature closure 174
presupposition
  53, 78, 98, 115, 116,
  132, 133, 141, 142,
  146, 155, 218
Pribram, Karl 3

Index   235

primacy 156, 174
projection 115, 130
proprioceptive sense 82
protocol 173
psychoneuroimmunology 62
punctuational ambiguity 220

quantum physicists 171

rapport
   12, 17, 20, 21, 42,
   43, 45, 170
reading 138
reality strategy
   44, 50, 51
recency 156, 174
recursion 181
refractory 17, 162
reframing
   69, 127, 135, 136,
   140, 158, 159, 216,
   225
Rehearsal Induction
   90, 91, 94
reintegration 118
REM 7
remedial work 122
repression 116
resource
   134, 146, 184, 185
revivification
   41, 42, 43, 45, 48,
   49, 54, 55, 58, 59,
   60, 67, 83, 110,
   116, 130, 142, 156,
   160, 191
rishi master 186
Robbins, Anthony 219
Rossi, Ernest
   7, 51, 52, 140

scope ambiguity 220
secondary gain
   106, 114, 136
self-appreciation
   149, 151, 158, 159,
   193

self-hypnosis 154
sensory acuity 137, 166
Sidis, Boris 16, 18, 20
sleep 79
slow wave sleep 155
somnambulism 10, 18
Spiegel, David 7
state-dependent 150, 155
storytelling 166
subjective referral 5
submodalities 106
sufficient trance 37
suggestibility 99
suggestion 140
surprise induction 85
symptom 136
synchronization 17
syntactic ambiguity 220

tag question 218
That's Right Exercise
   15, 33, 45
time distortion 106, 114
Time Line Therapy
   116, 160
tinnitus 140
TMJ muscles 217
tonality, voice 47
trance depth 19, 135
Transderivational Search
   (TDS) 85, 217
truisms
   52, 132, 133, 219
two minds 62, 67

ultradian rhythms 7, 37
unconscious mind
   2, 12, 21
universal examples
   105, 156
universal experiences
   104, 111
universal quantifier
   218, 222
unspecified verbs
   218, 222
uptime trance
   12, 36, 37, 38, 129
utilization 96

V-K Dissociation
   115, 216, 223
validation 143
Vedic scientists 171
Visual Squash 160
voice locus 117

waking state 67, 123
waking trance 19
waxy flexibility
   47, 82, 105
Wayne County Hospital
   22, 149
Weitzenhoffer, Andre
   6, 10, 16
well-formedness
   conditions
   131, 216, 224
Worcester State Hospital
   22

yoga 82

About The Authors

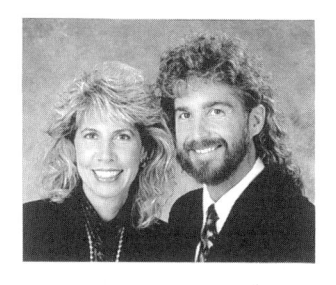

John Overdurf and Julie Silverthorn are highly respected international therapists and trainers of Hypnotherapy and NLP with over thirty years of combined experience. They are both Certified Master Trainers of NLP and the developers of Humanistic Neuro-Linguistic Psychology™, which integrates Hypnosis, Neurolinguistics, quantum theory, and spirituality.

They are completing their second book, *Dreaming Realities,* which outlines a psychological and spiritual system for using dreams for personal development. Married to one another for over sixteen years, they live their dream in the heart of Pennsylvania Dutch country with their cocker spaniel, Rio, and love every minute of it.

TRAINING AND RESOURCES

John Overdurf, C.A.C. and Julie Silverthorn, M.S. offer a wide variety of training and resources for personal and professional development.

HYPNOTHERAPY TRAINING

Hypnosis I
Two-day introductory training to traditional hypnosis as well as the methodology and wisdom of hypnotherapy pioneer, Milton H. Erickson, M.D.

Hypnosis II
Very popular advanced, four-day training in hypnotic approaches of Milton H. Erickson, M.D. that are the basis of *Training Trances*, as modeled by John and Julie.

HUMANISTIC NEURO-LINGUISTIC PSYCHOLOGY™ AND NLP TRAINING

NLP Practitioner Certification
7-day, tape-assisted home study
14 day comprehensive

NLP Master Practitioner Certification
8-day, tape-assisted flex track
14 day comprehensive

For more information on audio-tapes, books, trainings, resources, and personal coaching, call or write to:

Neuro-Energetics
111 Centerville Road
Lancaster, PA 17603

1-800-680-8803
(outside the USA)
1-717-293-8803

Metamorphous Press

Metamorphous Press is a publisher of books and other media providing resources for personal growth and positive change. MP publishes leading-edge ideas that help people strengthen their unique talents and discover that we are responsible for our own realities.

Many of our titles center around Neurolinguistic Programming (NLP). NLP is an exciting, practical, and powerful communication model that has been able to connect observable patterns of behavior and communication and the processes that underlie them.

Metamorphous Press provides selections in many useful subject areas such as communication, health and fitness, education, business and sales, therapy, selections for young persons, and other subjects of general and specific interest. Our products are available in fine bookstores around the world.

Our distributors for North America are:

Bookpeople	Moving Books	Pacific Pipeline
M.A.P.S.	New Leaf	the distributors
		Sage Book Distributors

For those of you overseas, we are distributed by:

Airlift (UK, Western Europe)
Specialist Publications (Australia)

New selections are added regularly and availability and prices change, so call for a current catalog or to be put on our mailing list. If you have difficulty finding our products in your favorite bookstore, or if you prefer to order by mail, we will be happy to make our books and other products available to you directly. Please call or write us at:

Metamorphous Press
P.O. Box 10616   Portland, OR   97210-0616
TEL (503) 228-4972
FAX (503) 223-9117

TOLL FREE ORDERING
1-800-937-7771

Metamorphous Advanced Product Services

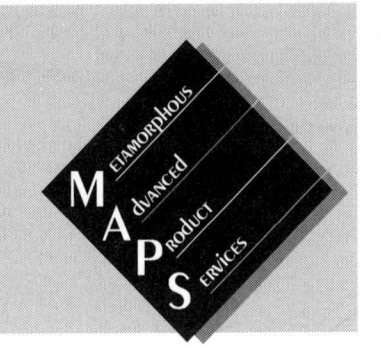

Metamorphous Advanced Product Services (M.A.P.S.) is the master distributor for Metamorphous Press and other fine publishers.

M.A.P.S. offers books, cassettes, videos, software, and miscellaneous products in the following subjects; Bodywork, Business & Sales; Children; Education; Enneagram; Health; (including Alexander Technique and Rolfing); Hypnosis; Personal Development; Psychology (including Neurolinguistic Programming); and Relationships/Sexuality.

If you cannot find our books at your favorite bookstore, you can order directly from M.A.P.S.

TO ORDER OR REQUEST A FREE CATALOG:

MAIL   M.A.P.S.
P.O. Box 10616
Portland, OR 97210-0616

FAX   (503) 223-9117

CALL   Toll free 1-800-937-7771

ALL OTHER BUSINESS:

CALL   (503) 228-4972